T0227629

Blocks and Freedoms in Sexual Life

A Handbook of Psychosexual Medicine

Ruth Skrine MBChB, MRCGP
Member of the Institute of Psychosexual Medicine

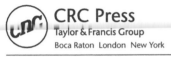

CRC Press
Taylor & Francis Group
Boca Raton London New York

CRC Press is an imprint of the
Taylor & Francis Group, an **informa** business

Contents

Acknowledgements

I would like to thank all those members and associates of the Institute of Psychosexual Medicine who have shared their work with me, especially those who have allowed me to use some of their clinical work in this book. In particular I want to mention the following who have given me encouragement, support and useful suggestions on earlier drafts: Tessa Crowley, Heather Montford, Roseanna Pollen, Robina Thexton and Prue Tunnadine.

Although my ideas and understanding have developed as a result of discussion with colleagues, the views expressed here are my own and do not represent those of the Institute or any other organization.

The names in this book are fictitious and personal details of patients have been altered to ensure anonymity. These include facts such as age, marital and social status and occupation. In addition the identity of the doctor in each case history is not disclosed. If any readers believe that they can recognize themselves in the histories, it is likely that they are identifying with aspects of someone else's story. In any event they can rest assured that no-one else will be able to recognize them.

Doctors interested in psychosexual medicine training may contact The Director of Training, Institute of Psychosexual Medicine, 11 Chandos Street, London WIM 9DE (Tel: 0171 580 0631).

Reprinted 2005

Radcliffe Publishing Ltd
18 Marcham Road, Abingdon, Oxon OX14 1AA, UK

British Library Cataloguing in Publication Data

A catalogue record for this book is available from the British Library.

ISBN 1 85775 159 0

Library of Congress Cataloging-in-Publication Data is available.

Typeset by Advance Typesetting Ltd, Oxfordshire
Printed and bound by TJI Digital, Padstow, Cornwall

With thanks to
Dr Iain Dresser
who helped me find some freedoms

Part I
Aspects of Doctoring

A psychosexual body/mind approach

Truth ... is a reality that exists in between two people seeking it ... truth can be seen or glimpsed, not possessed.

Neville Symington[1]

Sexual activity is dependent on both physical and emotional factors. The nerves, arteries and veins to the genital organs, not to mention the hormones throughout the body, need to be working adequately. At the same time, as anyone who has ever felt the stirring of sexual arousal within themselves will know, an almost limitless expanse of emotions can enhance or subdue arousal and sexual activity. Even to be able to masturbate with any degree of pleasure and satisfaction requires, for most individuals, appropriate physical stimulation combined with some particular thoughts and images that work in an erotic way for them.

This book is concerned with the search for some truths between the body and the mind. Since the time of Descartes these two aspects of man have been seen as separate. The ills of the two parts have been attended by different medical specialists, although general practitioners have always tried to care for the whole person. It is a difficult task, as the thinking processes of all of us have been channelled into the divide for so long that many doctors and patients still see an illness as 'real' or 'all in the mind'.

The term 'psychosexual medicine' is used by different people to describe different ways of working, each of which may have a different emphasis. In Britain since 1974 it has been used by the Institute of Psychosexual Medicine to describe an approach to sexual difficulties that attempts to take account of both sides of the Cartesian divide. The members of the Institute, originally mostly women doctors working in family planning clinics, and one psychoanalyst, Dr Tom Main, chose the term as a label for the skills they were trying to develop to help people who came to them with sexual problems.

The setting in which the term is used is important to the understanding of the viewpoint from which this book is written. It is based on my own clinical experience, and that of my colleagues in the Institute of Psychosexual Medicine, and is therefore enlightened and circumscribed by that experience. Any insights we have gained are based on our work with people who chose to bring their problem to a doctor, or other worker who deals with the body, and will therefore be different from those gained by, for example, a marriage guidance counsellor, psychoanalyst or priest, although there will, of course, be many overlapping areas. The skills and insights we have acquired are now used by doctors and others working in different settings, but their development at that particular time was at least in part an outcome of the contingency of the setting.

Most of our patients were not suffering from any illness, either physical or mental, but were healthy people who had come for contraceptive advice. Behind this overt request there were often anxieties and physical and emotional pains. We, the doctors and nurses, were freed from the pressure and responsibility of providing acute medical care, yet we were faced with distressed people for whom we felt we had little to offer. Our search for further training and understanding grew not from some particular interest in sexual matters (such interest was probably neither more nor less than that of any other group of people), but from the sense of hopelessness in the face of patients in need.

Now that most general practitioners are offering a comprehensive family planning service to their patients, it is in that setting that sexual difficulties are most often presented. This change is reflected by the sorts of doctor who are seeking further training with the Institute of Psychosexual Medicine. In 1988 two-thirds of the doctors in training worked in community medicine and one-third in general practice. In 1995 an equal number worked in general practice, the community and hospital medicine, mainly in gynaecology or genitourinary medicine. The presence of those working in hospitals is a sign of the increasing realization that sexual problems often present with physical complaints.

The method of training and study that we used, and that is still used, is based on the seminar method devised by Dr Michael Balint.[2] We were not provided with answers or theories, but with an opportunity to develop our skills. Thus for most of us the sense of not knowing what to do or how to help continued, but we gradually began to be able to tolerate such confusion with less despair.

Doctors are traditionally expected to have the answers or at least to be able to offer a view informed by knowledge and experience, and in many situations they can do just that. When it is a question of which antibiotic to use, or whether the patient needs to have an operation, such a view is worth canvassing and worthy of careful consideration. When the question is one of

'Should I leave my wife?' or 'Why have I gone off sex?', the doctor's view is not so useful because the answer lies within the person asking the question. Yet that person has not been able to find the answer alone and has chosen to come to a doctor for help. Often he has chosen a particular sort of doctor, a general practitioner whom he knows to be approachable about personal matters, a family planning or genitourinary doctor whose specialty implies an acceptance of sexual matters, or sometimes a newcomer or locum in a practice who has the advantage of being a stranger who need not be seen again. Help may be possible if the answer can be to allowed to 'emerge between' the patient and doctor during the consultation. Thus it has been necessary to develop some skills in working in a psychodynamic way, which is very different from the traditional role of the doctor as expert adviser or even caring counsellor and friend.

However, doctors have knowledge about and some responsibility for the bodies of their patients, and that cannot be ignored in their attempt to work differently with the patient's feelings. A simple example would be of a woman complaining that sex was painful. As in the case of headache, another very common but often baffling symptom, there may be many underlying causes, ranging from serious life-threatening disease such as a brain tumour to tension due to a row at home. Painful sex can be due to serious pelvic pathology, to an attack of thrush or to vaginal dryness from poor sexual technique, to name but a few possibilities. On the other hand, it may be due to emotional blocks to arousal. The doctor who develops psychodynamic skills but who wishes to remain someone who treats the whole person cannot forget his traditional physical doctoring, and it is this combination of emotional and physical interest and concern that provides the possibility of looking at the way in which the body and mind work together.

Such an approach is still far from common among doctors, and indeed often not expected or understood by those wanting help. Many men suffering from impotence will subject themselves to physical treatments, injections or operations, believing that their problem lies in their penis. Physical treatments of this kind can be very useful if there are serious physical disabilities causing the erectile difficulty. They can also have a powerful effect in combating anxiety, which is a major factor in all sexual problems, and in restoring confidence. Other men, however, have the sneaking feeling that perhaps that is not the whole story and look for other types of help.

Because sex is such a complicated activity, it can be difficult to begin to sort out the causes of problems, which may be partly physical and partly emotional. For example, we know that the mechanism of erection requires the veins of the penis to be able to retain the extra blood in it. Sometimes impotence can be caused by a venous leak, but the many complicated and deep emotions that are almost certain to be present in the person attached to that penis make a simple physical diagnosis fraught with difficulty. One might approach the problem by asking a back-to-front question. What degree of venous leak might be compatible with an erection adequate for intercourse in a sexually confident man in the presence of an interested woman whom he finds highly desirable and who makes him feel neither anxious, angry nor guilty? Such a question is, of course, impossible to answer, as those emotions can occur at all levels of the personality, including the deeply unconscious, and can never be completely understood or quantified.

The acceptance that we can never have complete answers or grasp the whole truth does not make the search a useless one. In my experience most patients are much more realistic about what doctors might be able to do for them than are the doctors themselves, who sometimes feel that they should be able to cure everyone of everything. I am not denying the hope that a magic answer can be found to a problem that is brought to doctors with differing degrees of urgency and pressure. 'You must do something doctor' does not necessarily mean that the patient believes you can, only that he wishes to impress on you the desperation of his case. If the desperation can be recognized in such a way that the person feels you are on his side, above all that you understand something of what it feels like to be him in his situation, it may be possible to begin to work together to search for a degree of understanding.

Case Study 1

Mr Abbot had seen many doctors to try to get help with his impotence of 8 years' standing. He had waited several months to see the psychosexual doctor and entered the room saying, 'Well, I hope you can help me because if I am not better in the next 6 months I am going to have a penile implant.' The doctor's heart sank, as it did not appear from the referral letter that Mr Abbot had any gross physical disease that might justify such a radical step. (The use of an implant requires the destruction of any natural erectile tissue that is present.)

Patient and doctor talked with difficulty about Mr Abbot's fury with all the doctors who had not helped him, including his feeling about having to wait so long for this appointment. Towards the end of the interview they were able to share something of his misery and despair at having lost a part of himself that was so precious.

As Mr Abbot left, the doctor asked whether he would like to come again, admitting that he did not have any magic and could not promise a cure in 6 months, or indeed at all, but that they could talk and try to understand it a bit together. The patient gave a charming smile and said he had not expected to be cured anyway, and yes, he would like to talk again.

The lack of sexual happiness, or at least 'good enough sex', which could be compared to Winnicott's 'good enough mothering',[3] causes much suffering both to individuals and to families, and that suffering can be damaging to health. Doctors and health care workers should therefore be among those many groups of people (not least friends, neighbours and relatives) who give thought to the problems. It is the fruit of some of that thinking that I am trying to capture here.

In medicine the place to begin is usually with a consideration of aetiology, the causes of things. I have already indicated that the causes of sexual difficulties often lie in both the body *and* the mind. There are further ways of trying to understand the emotional side, which I have summarized in an abridged form in Table 1.1.

What we believe about aetiology will affect what help is offered and in what way people feel they want to be helped. I believe that all the views listed in the table have some validity. In Chapter 3 I will look briefly at ideas about the structure of the personality, and it will become clear that many of the basic facts of our sexuality are determined early in life. However, there is ample evidence to show that subsequent experiences can also have damaging or enhancing effects on that part of our lives. A behavioural view holds that early sexual experiences under less than ideal conditions, in the back of a car or behind the bicycle shed for example, can produce a conditioned response such as premature ejaculation. That may be the case, but as I will show in later chapters other deeper emotions can often underlie what appears to be a simple symptom.

There is a widespread belief that sex is always about the relationship between the couple, and some doctors insist on referring couples to a

Table 1.1:   Aetiological views of sexual problems

Psychoanalytic
Behavioural
Sex as part of a relationship
Psychosexual: body/mind together

Table 1.2:   Skills of psychosexual doctoring

Listening; patient-centred consultation
Giving advice appropriately
Using reassurance sparingly
Tolerating not knowing what to do
Psychosexual genital examination
Use of the doctor–patient relationship

psychosexual clinic when individuals wish to come on their own. Such a belief seems to be a legacy of early behavioural sex therapy in which the method depended on both members of the couple being involved in the treatment. Of course, the relationship is a vital area for study, but it does not address the feelings that individuals have inside themselves and in relation to their own bodies.

As this book draws on the particular experiences of body/mind doctoring, I will not be dealing in detail with the other approaches listed. However, there is much overlap between them all, and we will not get anywhere near a realistic understanding if we stick rigidly to one aetiological belief. Where possible and where it seems appropriate, I will give reference to the other views.

Meanwhile I must return to my task of trying to explain what is meant by a psychosexual approach. One way of trying to convey a sense, a gut feeling, a taste of what such a view might be, is to describe the skills that doctors, nurses and others are working to develop in order to try to help (Table 1.2). Lists create artificially hard borders and boundaries, yet they can form a focus from which one can explore surrounding areas. The last two items in Table 1.2 are so important that I will devote a separate chapter to each of them. Here I will enlarge briefly on the other skills. The list is by no means comprehensive, and it includes aspects of the medical consultation that have been to some extent examined and analysed by other people. I have included these aspects in order to try to create a link with the sort of training and skills that are now being used in undergraduate and immediate post-graduate medical training.

Listening

If one tries to define listening, the meaning seems to become blurred and indistinct round the edges. At its simplest, we may know something has been said yet realize we have not heard the words. We may have to say, 'Could you repeat that? I didn't quite hear what you said', or more honestly, 'I'm afraid I stopped listening.' Yet there is more to listen to than words. The nuances of opening remarks, non-verbal communication and listening to what is not being said have all been discussed in texts about the consultation, such as that by Neighbour.[4] But where does listening overlap with feeling and lead on to thinking? The relationship between the last two is discussed later, but for now we can look at the effect of listening on the patient. How can we act so that the patient feels 'heard'?

For most people, despite the great openness about sexual matters in the media, their own sexuality is still a private matter. It is often easier to find a 'calling card' in the way of a symptom than to expose one's vulnerable sexual anxieties and inadequacies, which is one reason why it may be easier to go to a doctor with a physical complaint than to a counsellor or therapist, where an emotional difficulty has to be presented in all its nakedness.

Some sex therapists believe that it is important to take a sexual history by means of questions. Such an approach does show that the therapist is not afraid of using words to discuss the raw detail of sexual activity and to demonstrate that such discussion is allowable, but its cost is that of having a doctor (therapist)-led interview. It also deprives the patient of the opportunity to choose the starting place, and the doctor of the chance to begin to 'listen' with all his senses.

Such a listening does not mean blankness or necessarily silence but a focused attention, so that if the patient finds it difficult to begin to talk, that can be acknowledged and shared. Of course, there will be questions that spring to mind, but they will grow naturally out of the material that is being presented. They can then have the dual effect of eliciting information while at the same time making the patient feel he has had one's attention, as the question will be related to what he is saying rather than to the doctor's pre-conceived ideas.

The question that springs to mind is often better voiced in the form of a comment. 'I don't seem to have heard anything about your mother' notices her absence rather than demands her presence. The reply is more likely to throw light on why she has been absent, and to give some clue as to what she might mean to the patient.

Thus listening is an active attention that gives space and time for the story to emerge in its own way. Surprisingly, the time taken may be much less than that used up in routine history-taking. The doctor can help this birth by noticing and possibly commenting on the overt feelings, the half-hidden hints and gaps, so that the patient can gradually begin to believe that there is some under-standing of how he feels and to develop some trust that the doctor is on his side.

Freud has said that 'Listening is informed by forgetting'.[5] Of course, people need to know that their doctor remembers them as individuals and can remember details of their life, but an active memory of, for example, the last meeting with them can get in the way of listening now to the present trouble. In general practice I have sometimes been diverted by the last entry in the notes, wanting to know the outcome of that episode. The patient, however, has moved on and may even have forgotten about it completely. His or her mind is now fully occupied by the present problem, which needs to be heard. Bion expressed a similar idea by saying, 'What is required is a positive act of refraining from memory or desire'.[6] He is referring to the psychoanalyst, but I believe that there is something for the body/mind doctor to consider in his ideas. As I understand it, the desire, perhaps for one's own comprehension, therapeutic skill or cure for the patient, could interfere with keen listening in the same way as specific memories do. Adam Phillips[7] says, 'The analyst can catch the drift of the patient's unconscious...in the space cleared by relinquishing memory.' The ordinary doctor can perhaps hear better what the patient is trying to say if he can clear such a space, even if only for a brief moment.

Giving advice appropriately

I have already mentioned that advice is what is usually expected of a doctor, and that it is often right and proper that it should be given. The problem is that the advice needs to be based on evidence, traditionally collected by history-taking and examination, tests if necessary to make a differential diagnosis, and then the use of knowledge to advise on treatment and management. Such an approach has a very limited place in body/mind doctoring. If a definite physical diagnosis can be made, it will still be appropriate, as for example if there is evidence of some genital infection. When it comes to the more complicated area of feelings, the doctor is not in a position to give advice, as the evidence he or she has is always very limited.

However, because of the traditional roles of doctor and patient there is a pressure from both parties for the doctor to find the answers. Such pressure has to be consciously resisted. Instead the pressure needs to be understood and discussed, so that the focus of responsibility can shift, and the doctor and patient can become equal co-workers in their search for understanding. Such an approach is akin to that defined as counselling:

An interaction in which one person offers another person time, attention and respect with the intention of helping that person to explore, discover and clarify his way of living more resourcefully and to his greater well-being.

British Association for Counselling

Psychosexual medicine has tried to distance itself from counselling because of the very different expectations and setting for doctors and their patients compared with those for counsellors and their clients. However, I believe that at this point, when trying to break out of a traditional advice-giving role, it can be helpful to value and learn what we can from other traditions. I hope too that this book will help some non-medical counsellors and therapists to feel more comfortable with the body and the bodily pains of their clients. Although they do not have the opportunities of the physical examination, it may be possible for them to talk more freely about the body, and thus throw some links across the body/mind divide.

Using reassurance sparingly

Giving reassurance is another traditional thing doctors do, and patients certainly expect or hope for it. Like advice-giving, it may well be appropriate when the anxiety is unfounded and the doctor can use his greater knowledge honestly to put the anxiety to rest. In the psychosexual field the problem is to get to the root of the anxiety. Sometimes the patient knows what is worrying her, or him, but cannot find a way of telling the doctor. One example could be the young woman who comes to a doctor saying she is worried that something is wrong 'down below'. The doctor examines her and tells her that everything is normal. She still looks worried. If he had explored the specific worry, he might have found out that she had noticed that one side was bigger and hung lower than the other. Again, his reassurance that many women are not completely symmetrical and that she is normal does not relieve the worried look on her face. If he could have listened a bit longer, she might have found some way of admitting her fear that she had damaged herself by masturbating. Now they are in the area of an underlying anxiety.

Sometimes the causes of the anxiety are less conscious and may not be known to doctor or patient until they are expressed or felt in the consultation. I am not referring here to those deeply unconscious worries with their roots in the distant past that are the realm of the psychoanalyst, but to the worries that may suddenly emerge when working with a body/mind doctor. Some present anxieties are so disturbing that they are suppressed or 'forgotten' for the moment but can be recalled in a trusting relationship where the patient feels supported, understood and valued.

Case Study 2

Miss Brooks was complaining of painful intercourse. She had been examined by her doctor and by a gynaecologist and told she was quite normal. The problem continued and she came to see a psychosexual doctor. She began by talking about her relationship, which was going through a sticky patch because she wanted to buy a house but her boyfriend wanted to move away. She also mentioned that her sister had cysts of the ovary.

When, during a vaginal examination, the doctor refrained from talking but watched her face in an enquiring way, she suddenly asked about a lump in the vagina. The doctor could feel a perfectly normal cervix but nothing else, and asked how she knew about the lump. She said that she had felt inside for the first time when the pain started (possibly due to dryness or thrush at that time) and had found the lump. She had immediately connected it to her sister's problems, and now with the support of a listening doctor she could allow herself to feel and say that she was sure she had 'cancerous cysts'.

It seems that the idea that she had cancer was so frightening that she had suppressed it and allowed herself to be reassured, only to have the worry continue in an unstated form, showing itself as a continuing physical pain.

It has been suggested that the main effect of reassurance is to reassure the doctor, and it certainly gives one something to do when there does not seem to be anything else. For the patient reassurance can feel like a denial of the problem and is a powerful force in the process of making the patient feel misunderstood. I remember once telling a patient that there were lots of other people with a problem like hers, and she replied, banging the table, 'I'm not lots of other people, I'm me.' Sometimes, of course, it can be encouraging to feel you are not the only one with a problem, but if someone wants to know this, they will usually ask. Again, recognizing the anxiety behind the question may be more important than answering it. 'It seems you are afraid you may be different from other people' may add depth to a simple factual reply and can lead to further understanding of that person. My patient above knew she was different, and her anger was because she was not being appreciated as the individual she knew she was.

There is a danger in taking questions at face value, especially in the sexual field, where there is often so much embarrassment. Behind every general question asked in a professional setting is a personal anxiety. Until the details of the underlying anxiety have been explored, reassurance will be of very little help.

Tolerating not knowing what to do

The sense of being ignorant with the patient is a very new one for most doctors and tends to make us feel useless. We are the ones who are supposed to know, to be able to treat, to give advice and to reassure, to make our patients better. In this respect nurses and counsellors may have the advantage of being seen as comforters and carers rather than being expected to cure. Yet in other fields of medicine doctors have learnt to accept that they cannot always cure people, and much as we want to feel needed and useful, we have to learn to accept our limitations. The old adage is as true for psychosexual medicine as for any other branch. We can 'Cure sometimes, relieve often, comfort always', but we cannot offer comfort unless we are somewhere near the painful feelings. Sexual unhappiness is very painful and made worse by the fact that it is so often borne in secret.

The idea that we have to live with the experience of not having answers may suggest that there is nothing we can do in the face of sexual unhappiness. Nothing could be further from the truth. Body/mind doctors have a unique opportunity to study the way in which the mind and body react on each other. Psychosomatic medicine is often discussed in relation to the deepest levels of the person and to those illnesses which are thought to have unconscious causes requiring prolonged psychoanalysis. Our experience as psychosexual doctors suggests that many people are in a muddle about their minds and bodies at a much more easily accessible level, and that at times most ordinary people are at risk of feeling their pain in the wrong part of themselves.

Before leaving this introductory chapter it might be useful to look at the dilemma for the doctor faced with a patient complaining of a sexual difficulty. As in all branches of medicine, he or she has to make a differential diagnosis and decide on further action. Using the skills outlined above, many of which the modern general practitioner will have acquired during his vocational training, he might ask himself some of the questions listed in Table 1.3 and follow the suggested referral paths.

It is my hope that more general practitioners will increase their skills so that fewer referrals will be necessary. Sexual problems are so widespread that

Table 1.3:   Differential diagnosis/referral

Does the patient want or need to be referred?

1   Is the sexual problem part of a major psychiatric illness? ———➤ Psychiatrist

2   Is the sexual problem felt to be part of a marital problem? ———➤ Relate/marriage
    guidance

3   Are there long-standing personality problems or damage? ———➤ Social services/
    psychologist/self-help group

4   Is there a focused psychosexual problem in someone with a reasonably stable
    personality? If so, brief psychosexual work offered by the doctor himself, or
    ———➤ Psychosexual clinic
    Especially suitable for:
        Problems related to childbirth
        Problems related to abnormal smears
        Problems related to body fantasies
        Problems associated with physical symptoms
        Vaginismus
        Sexual symptoms that the patient wants to discuss with a doctor

Criteria
1   The patient must want to come
2   The patient must know what is on offer, i.e. discussion with a doctor who is
    interested in feelings, and also in the body, which he or she might suggest should
    be examined

---

there will never be enough 'specialists' to cope with the need. More importantly, many people do not want to be referred anywhere but wish to discuss
their pains with, and have their anxieties listened to by, the doctor of their
choice. Unless the patient is asking for referral it may be useful to see him or
her on at least two occasions, as although the doctor may feel that he has not
done very much, matters may seem very different to the patient after they have
been discussed.

Perhaps the most important reason why doctors should increase their
skills is the intertwined nature of bodily and emotional pains. Much unneces-
sary physical treatment, including some surgical intervention, could be
prevented if the skills of body/mind doctoring were more widespread, with a
consequent saving of pain for the patient and money for the community.

In the next two chapters I will look at two further skills that can be used
to provide understanding and relief for at least some of those people in distress.

References

1 Symington N (1986) *The Analytic Experience.* Free Association Books, London.

2 Balint M (1957) *The Doctor, his Patient and the Illness.* Pitman Medical, London.

3 Winnicott D W (1965) *The Maturational Process and the Facilitating Environment.* Hogarth Press, London.

4 Neighbour R (1987) *The Inner Consultation.* Petroc Press, Newbury, Berks.

5 Freud S, quoted in Phillips A (1994) *On Flirtation.* Faber and Faber, London.

6 Bion W (1970) *Attention and Interpretation.* Tavistock, London.

7 Phillips A (1994) *On Flirtation.* Faber and Faber, London.

2

The physical examination

Freud ... while working with Charcot, shifted the analyst's attention from looking to listening ... In effect, the body was dispersed, made invisible, with the invention of the talking cure.

Mary Kelly, artist[1]

Doctors have a long tradition of being licensed to examine and handle their patients' bodies. Indeed, they are not just licensed but in many situations have a duty to examine, so that they would be negligent in their professional work if they did not do so. They are, of course, not the only group of people who use touch for both diagnosis and treatment. It is not just those professionals who spring immediately to mind, such as nurses and physiotherapists, but also those working in osteopathy, using acupuncture or massage. This burgeoning army of helpers and healers also have licence to touch their patients or clients. However, the licence for doctors is most far-reaching in that it includes feeling and looking inside the body orifices and cutting into the body during surgical procedures.

Allowing another person to feel and manipulate one's body demands a degree of trust. Even the act of having a blood pressure check can be clouded by anxiety. What will happen? What will it feel like? Will he blow it up too tightly? Will she leave it on too long? Will I make a silly fuss? Already there is an inequality of power, a 'doer' and a 'done-to'. The patient begins to feel vulnerable.

When the examination is of more intimate parts of the body, the vulnerability is greatly increased. As the clothes come off and the body becomes more naked and exposed, so do the feelings. The natural reaction is to pull the couch blanket up to one's chin and compose one's features into a bright smile, or to fix one's eyes on the ceiling with detachment. For some the curiosity of what is happening and what the doctor is finding can overcome the sense of exposure, and the examination may then be a voyage of joint discovery.

For many there is an additional fear of what may be found, and the face of the doctor is searched for the smallest change of expression. Is there a lump? Is it cancer? Have I got AIDS? Is everything all right? It may be that the doctor cannot answer such questions immediately or conclusively, and the tension of unasked and unanswerable questions has to be borne by both people. Such tension may mask, reduce or increase the embarrassment for doctor and patient. There is a potential for embarrassment during all such intimate procedures, but the degree and the meaning of such feelings are very different on different occasions.

Both patient and doctor may fear their personal feelings in such an exposed position. As a young female doctor, I blushed easily and did not want to embarrass the adolescent boys I had to examine for their school medicals. Even the fear of blushing can bring a blush, so I developed a system whereby I examined the front of the body, including the genitals, and then quickly turned to the back to listen with my stethoscope. That way if there was a blush, it was hidden from my patient, and I could listen intently until it subsided.

Doctors have evolved a number of techniques to try to reduce such un-ease: the studious look with the avoidance of eye contact, bright conversation about the family or holidays, or a detailed description of what is being done and why. There is something to be said for these defences, and patients may be grateful for such distractions. For the doctor too it can be useful, as it is often difficult to be sure of what one is feeling or what the significance might be of anything felt. One needs time to think of the possibilities, the next move ... more questions? more tests? 'Get dressed and we'll have a chat' may be an appropriate response, especially if there is a strong possibility that there is serious disease present. However, such an approach denies the possibility of a further aspect of the examination.

Doctors working in psychosexual medicine use another dimension of the physical examination. It has been found that people in this vulnerable and exposed position sometimes blurt out things that surprise not just the doctor, but themselves as well. It is as if the removal of clothes removes a defence, a wall, a barrier that has prevented them saying something, or even letting themselves feel it. In order for this barrier to be lowered, the doctor needs to allow space and to be aware of his patient as a whole person. The effect is particularly marked when the genitals are being examined, when it has been called 'the psychosomatic genital examination', but it can occur during the examination of other parts of the body as well. Because of the depth and importance of the feelings that may emerge, it has been described as 'the moment of truth'.[2]

There has been, and still is, a great deal of misunderstanding about this concept. It can be seen as an attempt on the part of the doctor to 'pry into secrets'. I was once asked whether I obtained a patient's consent to do a psychosomatic examination, as if it was some extra invasive technique that was being used 'on' the patient. It is nothing of the kind. It is no more than a heightened awareness, a more concentrated listening to spoken and unspoken communications, during an examination that has a genuine physical content and justification. It is an enabling moment for patients who may be able to get in touch with feelings they did not know they had.

I must digress for a moment to express my concern at the idea, suggested and put into practice in some places, that the genital examination should be used by non-doctors as an adjunct to other therapies. Such an idea is, I believe, profoundly wrong. The approach is not a new 'tool' like an X-ray machine; it is a sensitization of a particular moment in a relationship. The history of the relationship between doctors and patients goes back a long way and involves a great deal of trust that is partly built on that history. Of course, there are clumsy doctors, hurtful doctors, untrustworthy doctors; we are, after all, fallible members of the human race. Perhaps all of us are some of those things some of the time. But despite that fact, most people who chose to come to us do so because they trust us to some extent. There is a background of expectation on both sides that lies behind the idea of licence to examine, which includes the assumption that the examination is in the patient's best interest.

Such expectations cannot be easily transferred to other workers, despite careful explanation. Even doctors working in different settings have to be very clear about what licence they have and what expectations are present on both sides. For example, some psychiatrists still see themselves as whole-person doctors, able to examine for and treat physical disease. However, many patients expect such doctors to be interested only in their minds, so that the suggestion of a physical examination of any kind could be felt as an intrusion or even an assault. Such a misunderstanding can also occur if an ordinary body doctor such as a general practitioner is seen as wearing a 'counselling' hat, when again the patient might expect a 'talking' treatment rather than a physical one.[3]

There is a possibility that such a claim to special licence will be seen as another example of doctors trying to claim special privilege, or that they are trying to keep some magic to themselves. This is perhaps partly the fault of those of us who have had the experience of the almost magical contact and empathy that can occur at such moments. It is easy to exaggerate the power and to deny the possible dangers and limitations. The setting in which each of us works, whether we are counsellors, psychoanalysts, priests or doctors, affects the opportunities and limitations of what we have to offer. I do not think we serve others best if we deny the differences and fail to examine the strengths and weaknesses of each approach. This is not to say that we should not learn what we can of each other's disciplines and use what can be used, but any skill will be different when transported to a different setting. 'The cobbler should stick to his last' is not a bad motto for those in the helping professions, although we can get ideas about the type of last we use from studying other people's models.

Returning to the body/mind doctor who is trying to treat the patient as a whole person, there will often come a time, during the course of a routine medical consultation, when there is an opportunity to examine the patient.

Case Study 3

Miss Evans was a young woman who came to a family planning clinic to have her vaginal diaphragm checked. She mentioned during the preliminary discussion that she could not get an orgasm. It was clear that she was able to become aroused during intercourse, but she could not let herself go any further. Discussion did not seem to uncover any specific fear, but during a routine check of her diaphragm she appeared rather giggly. The doctor commented that she seemed to find it a bit embarrassing, and wondered if it were perhaps like that when she made love. The patient clamped her hand over her mouth and said, 'Oh, I am so afraid that I might cry out and make a silly noise.' Following the examination, the patient talked for a few more minutes about how she needed to be 'sensible' in order to win her parents' approval. Her younger sister was the exciting, scatterbrained, silly one, and she had to be the opposite if she were to be valued by her parents. Having shared the feeling of silliness with a doctor who could also value her as a reasonable person, she became orgasmic before her next visit.

Every intimate examination can reveal something about the whole person, but because of the revelatory nature of some such encounters, less dramatic evidence may be ignored or undervalued. A woman who appears relaxed and easy within the clinical setting may be showing that she is comfortable with her own body and can trust the doctor to do whatever is necessary within that setting. Others who appear to cut off from the process of examination may be frightened and mistrustful of doctors, or they may have a mistrust of their own bodies. A comment that it seems very uncomfortable for them may be answered by 'I hate examinations' (no-one *likes* them). In some instances it is possible to enquire whether they are like this with their partner. It may well be that there are no problems in the privacy of their own lives and that it is just the exposure in the clinical situation that is so difficult.

Sometimes the intimacy of the moment can allow the sharing of painful and personal emotions, especially if the patient already senses that the doctor has some understanding of, and sympathy with, his or her internal feelings. The exploration has to be carried out tentatively and with sensitivity. The idea of a safe, shared space between the internal worlds of doctor and patient is a useful one.[4] Within such a space patients may discover something that they did not know they felt, or make connections between different parts of themselves that help them to make sense of their feelings and pains, be they physical or emotional.

Case Study 4

Mrs Farrell complained that sex with her husband had become painful. They had been married for 4 years and there appeared to be no obvious physical or emotional change that had taken place at the time the pain had started, 6 months previously. It was not until the moment of vaginal examination that she said, 'I know and you know what the trouble is.' In fact the doctor had no idea, but in response to a questioning look the patient said, 'I am furious with him.' As she dressed and sat down she was quiet and thoughtful. Finally, she looked at the doctor and said, 'I realize I have to make some changes in my life.'

For Mrs Farrell the examination had allowed her to relocate her pain out of her vagina and into her unsatisfactory marriage. The examination had not been painful, but the doctor had watched her face and refrained from saying too much. In some way the absence of genital pain, but the presence of another person who was concerned with the pain wherever it might be, had allowed her to feel it in the appropriate part of herself. For some reason she had not been able to face her anger by herself, but once she had done so in the presence of the doctor, she was confident that she wished to deal with it in her own way without further help.

What can the doctor do to help these moments of discovery? It is, of course, important to provide privacy, warmth and the simple comforts of a blanket and a chair for clothes. The patient needs to know what part of the body you want to examine, but the way in which he or she responds may be interesting. If the examination couch is in the same room behind a screen or curtain, there is an opportunity for comments while dressing and undressing. 'I've always hated being examined' may be easier to say when hidden from the doctor. For some who have agreed to examination, the act of getting onto the couch is too difficult and they will be found sitting on the chair fully clothed, sometimes in anger, sometimes in terror.

Each of these moments is an opportunity for the doctor to try to understand, and to share with the patient, the blocks that are making it so difficult. In psychosexual work the discussion of the examination is often as important as the examination itself. Dr Perrin describes a situation where she put on a glove in preparation for a vaginal examination, but then, in response to the patient, she stood by the couch talking, and eventually took the glove off without ever touching the patient.[5] If the fear is of physical pain, the doctor must allow the patient to be in control, offering reassurance that the examination will go at her pace. This is particularly important when undertaking a vaginal examination if the complaint is of painful sex or an inability to consummate the relationship.

However, there are pitfalls in an 'oh so gentle' approach. The patient has come for help, and running away from her fear is unlikely to help. One must try and stay with it and explore the details of the fear while helping her to feel you are on her side. Doctors who can use their own feelings as diagnostic instruments may get some clues to the unconscious fear if they can pull out and study what is going on in themselves. This idea is explored further in the next chapter, but for now it may be worth asking whether the doctor feels a sense of being too powerful, almost an abuser or a rapist. Some patients send out strongly contradictory messages. Such messages may be spoken: 'Don't mind if I shout, I just want you to get on with it.' Others create a feeling of great conflict in the doctor, which may lead to a misjudgement that leaves the patient feeling as if he or she has been attacked. The internal boundaries have been violated and the doctor has stepped out of the shared, safe space. If the confusion within the doctor can be interpreted in such a way that the patient's ambivalence is discussed, it becomes safer to proceed together step by step.

Case Study 5

Mr Gibbons had never managed to have intercourse and felt that he had great difficulties relating to women. However, he told the doctor that he had once tried to make love to a woman. On that occasion the attempt had been followed by several days of swelling and soreness of his penis, enough perhaps to put off even a confident man. Discussion of this episode made him feel physically squeamish, and it was with reluctance that he got onto the couch to be examined. The female doctor found herself delaying the examination of the genitals by listening to the heart and chest for a long time. Finally, she said, 'May I look at the offending bits?', and managed to palpate the testicles and penis. The patient was uncircumcised, and she asked whether the foreskin went back all right, suggesting he might pull it back to show her. He said he had never done that and could not possibly do so. The doctor was tempted to do it for him, but she had a sense that to do so would be an attack on him, almost a rape. She shared the feeling and he said he would like to try to do it at home. With the doctor's encouragement he did indeed find the courage to do so, and began to feel more in touch with and confident about his own body.

One can surmise that Mr Gibbons must have had traumatic early experiences that had left him afraid of his own body, and afraid of the power of women over him. Such influences could not be explored in great depth or detail in a brief relationship, but by recognizing the conflict within herself, the doctor was able to offer him an experience of being with a woman who was in a position of potential power over his body, yet who could respect his autonomy.

The sense of confusion in the consulting room and within the doctor may mirror the confusion within the patient and in his personal relationships. If this confusion is present, the maintenance of the boundaries of the two selves becomes particularly important and difficult. The embarrassment that can develop in relation to the physical examination can be threatening to the personal boundaries of patient or doctor. In the following example the doctor felt she had to tread very carefully not to intrude into the patient's private and well-defended space in a way that might be destructive or overwhelming for him.

Case Study 6

Mr Holden complained that he had lost interest in sex. It was not till his third visit that he reluctantly agreed to let the doctor examine him. She explained (again) what sort of doctor she was and that physical examination would be part of her normal practice. He looked acutely embarrassed, and the doctor felt that to insist would be abusive. She found herself saying that he did not have to go through with it. 'Well, I want help and if that is what you have to offer it must be sensible for me to agree.' Some degree of trust had been established.

It was not until he was safely dressed and back in his chair that Mr Holden could tell the doctor that he had been afraid that he might get an erection. Now his anxiety was because he had not done so. He wanted to know what the doctor had expected? She replied that she had not anticipated such a thing but would not have been surprised or upset had it happened.

What an awful double-bind for this man, with his sense that to get an erection in a clinical situation would be an offence, yet not to do so might be seen as a weakness in himself or an affront to the femininity of the doctor. Out of the relief of being able to talk about it with a doctor who in this instance did not herself feel threatened, Mr Holden found himself able to share other details of his sexual life that had been burdening him and that he had so far not been able to broach. It is interesting that this included some confusion about the rectitude of sex with 'nice' women. It seems as if his confusion about whether he wanted an erection in the consulting room echoed his confusion about sex with respectable women.

I have heard it suggested at undergraduate level that students and doctors should never mention sex while examining a patient. Such a blanket prohibition shows great anxiety that the doctor might do something that could be construed by the patient as sexual. Such a safety precaution may be useful for the inexperienced doctor, but a more important skill is to listen to one's own reactions to the individual patient and try to understand them. For example, with Miss Evans, described above, the doctor felt quite comfortable referring to love-making while checking her diaphragm. With Mr Holden, however, neither doctor nor patient could mention sexual arousal until he had regained the safety of his clothes.

Such a feeling of comfort or discomfort does not necessarily depend on the actual sex of the doctor and patient. A sense of embarrassment and vulnerability can be present with a doctor of the same sex and may be even worse for some patients for all sorts of different reasons. For example, a woman may prefer a male doctor if she has had the experience of an invasive, all-powerful mother who tended to take over her body when she was a young child. Quite a large number of men prefer a woman doctor, perhaps because the competitive element is missing in the relationship. A man may find it easier to admit that he believes his penis to be too small if he does not feel that the doctor has one to compare it with. The presence of hidden homosexual feelings may be particularly difficult for the heterosexual doctor to recognize.

The doctor is not the only one who is anxious that the interview should not be sexualized. Patients want the help of doctors or they would not have come. If the interview develops sexual undertones, the doctor cannot do his job, whether that is discussing private matters or physically examining the patient. If the presence of sexual feelings can be silently recognized, whether they are being felt by the doctor or suspected to be occurring in the patient, and thought about as a clinical event, they will usually become defused.

A particularly useful concept is that the sexuality may be an unconscious defence used by the patient who fears what the doctor's work might uncover.[6] It may take the form of a flirtatious female patient with a male doctor, who makes it quite impossible for him to feel safe enough to perform an examination even with a chaperone present. Alternatively, a man may get a particularly threatening erection during examination by a female doctor. There may be situations in which such a demonstration of potency is more likely to occur, such as during a consultation for infertility, where the man may unconsciously need to demonstrate a potency that he feels is being questioned along with his fertility.[7]

On some occasions it is the doctor who may feel that her or his personal space has been invaded. Dr Crowley has written sensitively about the sense of being overwhelmed by a patient's pain when she allowed herself to feel too much of it.[4] On that occasion the doctor, during a physical examination, had made an intuitive guess about previous sexual abuse. The sense of violation that the doctor felt mirrored that felt by the patient.

Such a feeling is particularly upsetting if the invasion has been in the nature of an unspoken sexual threat. Again it can be helpful if such a feeling can be understood as an unconscious defence. However, doctors of both sexes will need to be sensitive to more disturbed patients who cannot accept the traditions of the clinical situation and who may try to use the doctor as a sexual object.

One of the advantages of the seminar method of training is that the subject of sex, an emotionally charged one for both patient and doctor, becomes a matter for clinical study and evaluation. The sexual tensions that inevitably develop from time to time within the consulting room can be viewed as clinical findings rather than professional or personal failures. The honest reporting of such events not only allows more work with the patient, but also reduces the possibility of sexual misconduct with patients. Such temptations will be less strong in brief or episodic encounters than in intense long-term therapy. I suspect also that they are less likely to occur in relationships with doctors, who are imbued with the professional constraints of the physical examination from the earliest days of their training, than with non-medical therapists. However, such things have been known to happen, and we should not underestimate what Rutter[8] calls 'the allure of the forbidden', with its catastrophic results for patient and doctor alike.

Considerations of confusion and conflict have led this discussion into an area of body/mind doctoring that raises great anxiety. Once such fears can be studied, and doctors can begin to allow some freedom into their thinking and feeling during the examination, it can become an opportunity for other discoveries. The feeling may not be a sense of conflict but more an idea or an image that forces itself into the doctor's consciousness.

Case Study 7

Mrs Jones came to the doctor because she had lost interest in sex since the birth of her daughter 6 years before. The birth had been physically very traumatic and Mrs Jones had developed a utero-vesicular fistula. After the birth she had passed urine through her vagina for several weeks until it was repaired. Since then she had urinated normally and had been reassured that all was normal. The doctor found a normal pelvis on examination, but suddenly had a strong feeling within herself that the two organs were still joined. She suggested to the patient that although she knew in her mind that these two organs were now separate, it did not feel as if they were actually separate within her own body. The patient cried with relief that her irrational but strong body feeling had been recognized. Perhaps it is not surprising that she could not reclaim her vagina for pleasurable sexual use if it still felt connected to her bladder.

Such moments of empathy are difficult to describe and cannot be forced. I suspect that the doctor picks up minimal clues that are not consciously understood. The ability to allow mental images to flood the mind, and then share them tentatively with the patient, provides a different tool in the doctor's armature. The offer must be tentative, for the image may have come from something within the doctor, but if so it will make no sense to the patient and can be rejected. In the following case the feeling was strong, and the interpretation seemed to make sense, but it may not have been enough to allow the patient to let go of his phantasy.

Case Study 8

Mr King had suffered from impotence for the last 8 years. He was a fit man in his early 40s, but his desperate wish for a cure had led him to try penile injections, pumps, hormones and two operations on the veins of his penis. Nothing had helped. As his female doctor examined his penis, he got the beginning of an erection but appeared totally disconnected from it. The doctor had a strong image of a cut across his middle, a line, an unbridge-able gap dividing his mind from his genitals. The line seemed to have been created by all the medical interference to which he had been subjected. (I am not here blaming those colleagues who were I believe acting in response to his desperation with the tools they had available to them.) Sharing the feeling of his total divide between his mind and his body, and the sense of an almost physical division between the two, seemed to allow the beginning of an acceptance that his mind could have some effect on his body and that it was not all a mechanical problem in his penis. How-ever, he had lived with the sense of this divide, and the hope that doctors would cure his body, without taking any responsibility for his own feelings for so long that the doctor was doubtful that the connection they began to make together would survive.

The doctor needs to be sensitized to his or her own sense of surprise when confronted by strange feelings or images. I remember once when taking a cervical smear from a woman who was terrified of all examinations that I looked in amazement at the spatula as I withdrew it. Somehow I expected it to be at least a foot and a half in length, and could not believe it was so short. As she looked at it the patient began to express her feeling that it had to go 'to my throat' and that she imagined her uterus to be the size of a football.

Every physical examination takes place within a relationship between two people. Ideas about the doctor–patient relationship will be discussed in the next chapter and are particularly relevant to the moment of the exam-ination, where the interactions are not only active, but may also be present in a particularly condensed or heightened form.

Recently, a woman patient of mine told me that her doctor had said of me, 'She will examine you and find out if you are frightened of sex.' What a travesty of the shared moment that I have been trying to explain. The anxiety or fear may well be about the examination rather than about sex. The feelings that are touched may be to do with the individual's fears or phantasies about his or her own body rather than anything connected with a sexual partner. Old experiences of being invaded by medical intervention or by previous abusive experiences, either physical or emotional, may be remembered or suppressed. Perhaps most surprisingly, the feelings may be far removed from sex or the genital area, related instead to deep emotions such as feelings of worthlessness, guilt, anger or grief.

In the following chapters I will explore some of these aspects of the whole person and the way in which they can contribute to the blockage of the free and joyful expression of sexuality. The physical examination, and the vulnerability that precedes and follows such an intimate moment, can provide an opportunity to make connections between the mind and the body, and in so doing begin to make sense of the pain that has brought the patient to the doctor. The causes of such pain may be physical, emotional or, in many cases, a mixture of both, so that a doctor who can think about the body and the mind together is in a good position to offer help.

References

1   Kelly M (1990) Re-presenting the Body. In *Psychoanalysis and Cultural Theory* (ed. J Donald), Macmillan, London.

2   Tunnadine P (1992) *Insights into Troubled Sexuality*. Chapman & Hall, London.

3   Freedman R (1995) On Being a 'Counsellor'. *Institute of Psychosexual Medicine Journal*. 9: 14.

4   Crowley T (1995) Seminar Training and the Development of Boundaries. *Institute of Psychosexual Medicine Journal*. 9: 6.

5   Perrin J (1996) Aspects of the Psychosomatic Examination. *Institute of Psychosexual Medicine Journal* 11: 10.

6   Skrine R (ed.) (1987) *Psychosexual Training and the Doctor/Patient Relationship*. Chapman & Hall, London.

7   Coulson C (1995) Expectations and Surprise: Thoughts in an infertility clinic. *Institute of Psychosexual Medicine Journal*. 9: 9.

8   Rutter P (1989) *Sex in the Forbidden Zone*. Unwin Hyman, London.

3

Psychodynamics and the doctor–patient relationship

There is a road from the eye to the heart that does not go through the intellect.

G K Chesterton[1]

We are thinking beings, and we cannot exclude the intellect from participating in any of our functions.

William James[2]

The term 'doctor–patient relationship' is perhaps an unfortunate one for the attitude of mind I am trying to describe. It suggests that there could be, for example, good or bad, close or distant, supportive or aggressive relationships, and that the first of each of these pairs is somehow better than the second. The meaning of the term as used here is different, with the focus on the study of the relationship and its use as a way to help the patient.

The aim is not to try to foster a particular relationship but to study what actually happens between two people from minute to minute. In order for this study to take place the doctor must be able to pull out, observe and think about not just his patient's responses, but his own as well. This idea is expressed in pictorial form by Neighbour (Figure 3.1). There is, as it were, a third person, a spectator at the feast. Such observations will be of no use unless there is a degree of real empathy between the doctor and patient, as the only way to begin to understand someone else's feelings is to feel some of them oneself. Yet it is impossible to think and feel at the same time, so the activity has to be one of going in and feeling and then pulling out and thinking. The Neighbour spectator in dotted outline suggests one who comes and goes many times during the consultation. The two quotations at the head of this chapter express something of the dynamic tension that the two activities can provoke.

In a highly developed form the spectator has been named by Casement the 'internal supervisor'.[3] Casement uses the term in relation to the psychotherapist, but the concept is one that can also be applied to other therapeutic

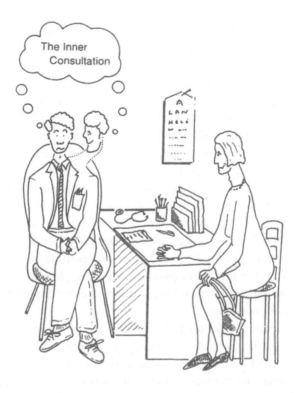

Figure 3.1:   The inner consultation. (Reproduced from Neighbour R, 1987, *The Inner Consultation*, Petroc Press, Newbury, Berks, with kind permission of the publisher and author.)

relationships. What is being watched is not just the patient or the doctor, but what is going on between them. What is the patient doing to the doctor, and what is the doctor doing to the patient? What sort of atmosphere are they creating together?[4]

Such self-questioning will be familiar to anyone who works in a psychodynamic way, and this way of thinking is the basis of psychodynamic psychotherapy. The skill is used at its highest level in psychoanalysis when the words 'transference' and 'countertransference' are used to describe some of the many feelings that arise and are passed between the couple in that setting. Transference is the word used to describe the way in which feelings towards someone from the past get transferred on to and felt towards the therapist who is present. Thus old, sometimes very old, feelings can be re-experienced. Countertransference is more complicated because it concerns feelings of the therapist towards the patient, and therefore is not only specific for that patient at that time, but also holds the potential of being influenced by feelings arising within the therapist that are personal to him or her.

Such technical words are sometimes used in a more general sense about the feelings that pass between people in any setting, or even between people and institutions, which can make their specific meaning in any particular instance hard to capture. A difference has been made between 'transference neurosis', that which develops during psychoanalysis, and transference in this more general sense. As has been discussed in the previous chapter, every meeting between a doctor and a patient carries unspoken assumptions about the relationship. It is therefore more accurate to refer to the doctor–patient relationship rather than to use the words transference and countertransference. It is also much more useful, as the particular advantages and disadvantages of that relationship, the possibilities and boundaries that it provides, can be explored. In the same way psychosexual work by nurses needs to be a study of the nurse–patient relationship, as that will carry different expectations, opportunities and limitations.

It takes time for the doctor to become aware of the interaction between himself and the patient, and to understand it in such a way as to illuminate the patient's problem. It is not easy to describe the study of this relationship on paper. However, the existence of the interaction is the essential theme of every clinical encounter used as an example in this book. The idea of studying the 'here and now' interaction between the doctor and the patient, as a way of understanding some of the unconscious feelings, has been borrowed from psychoanalysis. It could be argued that this approach uses a doctor who, not having been through a full personal analysis, is in some sense incompletely trained. However, the circumscribed scope of psychosexual medicine, and its differentiation from psychoanalysis, has been clearly stated,[5] and an appropriate group training method has been available for the past 20 years.[6]

The doctor trained in this way develops skills that can be used in comparatively brief contacts with patients, either during his routine work in surgery or clinic, or during a few rather longer interviews. The ability to observe what is going on during a physical examination has already been discussed. The information that can be gathered from noticing the atmosphere of the consultation can have direct relevance to the patient's problem.

Case Study 9

Mrs Clark went to her doctor complaining that she could no longer respond sexually to her husband. Having stated her problem, she sat and waited, looking calm and expectant. The doctor asked whether she could tell him a bit more about it, but she said, 'Not really. That is just it. I do not want to make love any more.' In the face of this cold composure, and feeling that he had to find the answers, the doctor started to ask questions, which were met with short, factual replies.

It had started at Christmas, all had been well before, she got on well with her husband, she could think of no change in her life. The questions became more pressing, until the doctor suddenly realized that in the face of the frigidity in the room he was becoming more and more active. At that point he said, 'It seems difficult for you to get in touch with any real feelings.' She became thoughtful, and it was as if for the first time they could both tolerate some silence in the room. Finally, she admitted that she did not find it easy to show her feelings, and they began to wonder together why that might be.

Enough rapport was established for Mrs Clark to agree to return, and at the next meeting she was able to remember that she had felt envious of her sister at Christmas when she had been playing with her baby. She and her husband had decided they were not yet ready for children, but now she could share her ambivalent feelings about the good job that she might have to give up and her growing wish for motherhood. After talking to the doctor, she was able to let out more of her feelings to her husband and as a result the sexual situation improved.

Although it can be very misleading to generalize about people, some patterns in the atmosphere that develops between a doctor and a patient with a sexual problem have emerged. For example, the impotent man may arouse irritation in the woman doctor who feels frustrated by an apparently compliant man who cannot show his anger or assert himself either in the consulting room or at home, yet defeats her and his partner by remaining passively impotent. A different feeling has been noticed in a study of men who could not ejaculate in the vagina.[7] Here, the women doctors tended to react to the patients with excitement and optimism at first, only to be finally disappointed. Such a feeling was often akin to that felt by the partners of these men.

More important than the recognition of patterns is the ability to think afresh on each occasion about the way in which the patient is treating the doctor and what reaction this is producing from moment to moment. In particular, because of the sexual focus of our work, it is possible to find evidence of the patient's concepts of his own sexuality by studying the relationship with the doctor, who is a sexed being. Some understanding of how he treats people of the same, or opposite, sex outside the consulting room can be gained. In long-term therapy the establishment of transference allows the therapist to take on the attributes of important people in the patient's past, whatever their sex. In brief body/mind doctoring the relationship of the patient to the reality of the sex of the doctor provides a different sort of evidence, and it may be possible to interpret that evidence to the patient.

Case Study 10

Mr Carey, an intelligent man, very successful in his large business, had never been able to make love to his wife of 3 years' standing. He saw his own sexual arousal as something rather gross and 'animal', although he could get good erections and enjoyment from masturbation using heterosexual phantasies. He talked easily and openly to the doctor about his life, telling her that his father had died when he was 13. He had two younger sisters and had felt the need to take over the role of head of the family.

   Several meetings took place, which appeared to be enjoyed by both doctor and patient. It was only gradually that the doctor noticed that she was becoming irritated by his concern for her health, and even his obsessive need to arrive not a minute early or a minute late, convenient though that was. Once the doctor had interpreted his need to treat her with such care, as if she were glass that might break if exposed to a more dynamic and assertive part of his manhood, they were able gradually to move forward.

One must accept that the doctor will have personal feelings that can affect the consultation, but he may be aware of some of them and they will not make him react in the same way to every patient. For example, the doctor who has had a row with his wife before coming to the surgery, and who arrives in surgery in a bad mood, may manage to keep his temper with seven patients, only to lose it with the eighth. Why? What was it about that particular patient that made him feel so angry? There may be something to be learnt that can be useful in trying to understand the patient's predicament. The feelings and actions of the doctor can thus become a clinical finding that may provide evidence of the way the patient is.

It is not only the doctor's feelings, but also his or her actions that can throw light on the problem.

Case Study 11

Mrs Carr had been married for 3 years and had not been able to consummate her marriage. She was a thin, frail-looking woman who made the doctor feel protective. One day the doctor found herself writing in her diary 'Mrs Carr. Don't be late.' She also found herself driving the patient home one day for no very obvious reason. Suddenly, she realized that this frail-looking waif was in fact very powerful and was controlling all those around her, including her doctor. Once this had been recognized it was possible to interpret her behaviour, not by attacking her for acting in this way, but by wondering with her what was so frightening about the idea of losing control. The patient was able to connect that remark to her fear of being damaged both emotionally and physically, and to the intense sense of fragility, especially in her vagina, which was being protected by muscle spasm.

The idea that what is going on in the consulting room can be a clinical event to be studied can be very freeing for the doctor because it removes the sense of 'Was that right or wrong?', and replaces it with 'What was the meaning of what happened?' Most doctors are very anxious to do the right thing and to help their patients as best they can, but this very wish can sometimes obscure their understanding. Situations may arise in which the doctor feels inadequate or even attacked by his patient, and unless that can be understood he or she may retaliate, leaving the patient in turn feeling misunderstood and attacked.

At this point it may be useful to look at another psychoanalytic concept, that of defence mechanisms. These defences occur at all levels of the personality of both doctor and patient. At a deeply unconscious level they defend the individual from overwhelming anxiety and spring from the earliest days and weeks of life. Such defences are essential, for as Anthony Storr says, 'no human being could possibly manage his life without defences of various kinds'.[8] The idea of defences can be a useful one for the body/mind doctor, not in order that they can be knocked down, but to help him to recognize that the feeling inside himself may be arising from the patient's need to defend inner areas of vulnerability. Such a defence may be felt as a withdrawal or even an attack. In the face of such a defensive attack the doctor is tempted to run away or attack in return. The task of recognizing the defence and staying with it by paying tribute to it is difficult, but this may allow patients gradually to reveal more of themselves.

The varieties of defence that have been described in psychotherapeutic work can all be seen in psychosexual medicine; these include denial, regression, projection and splitting, where good and bad feelings are separated in a variety of ways.[9] There are, of course, many other psychic ways of defending against pain, but in psychosexual medicine these are often accompanied by physical complaints that may be used as the presenting symptom. The following case shows how the patient dealt with painful feelings by projecting her anger onto the doctor and also unconsciously involving her body.

Case Study 12

Mrs Day complained of a numb feeling in her vagina that had been present since the birth of her baby 2 years previously. She was convinced that she had been 'stitched up wrong' in such a way that the nerves had not been reconnected. The doctor noticed the force of her anger (it would have been impossible not to!) and even found himself feeling personally responsible for the problem, even though he had not been involved in the delivery. Although he too began to feel angry with those who had charge of her care, there did not seem to have been any obvious negligence on the part of his colleagues, and he managed to refrain from colluding with her attack and from defending his colleagues. He was thus able to stay with her sense of being a victim without taking sides.

The doctor's observation was that the baby did not seem to feature in her talk at all. Gradually, over a series of four meetings, her anger subsided and she began to talk about how things were before the birth of the baby, and how much not just her body, but also her whole happy life had been changed. As the degree to which she felt changed by the baby became clearer, she was able to stop projecting her pain outwards and begin to feel what she had lost within herself. At the same time she was able to acknowledge how much she did in fact love the baby, and her sexual feelings began to return.

As well as being an example of defensive projection, this case illustrates the importance of listening to what is not being said. The open-ended consultation, in which the patient chose the subject matter, allowed the absence of the baby to be noticed. In the same way the ability to allow the patient to go back to the past only when and if she or he chooses to do so allows specific memories to surface, and these too will contain absences that can act as clues that have been compared to Sherlock Holmes' dog that 'did not bark in the night'.

Perhaps this would be a good place to consider briefly some of the other concepts that have so far been taken for granted by my use of terms such as 'unconscious' and 'levels of the personality'. As I have already indicated, I am convinced that our sexual feelings spring from the deepest parts of our personalities and are shaped and affected by all our experiences from the earliest hours and days of our existence up to the present time. Indeed, it is likely that our genetic make-up and our prenatal experiences also play a part in our sexual functioning, although it is very difficult to untangle the earliest experiences from the given make-up of any individual.

We could perhaps compare this structure which is ourselves to a building. The soil and subsoil on which the building stands is a physical given, as is our genetic nature. The man-made foundations can be compared with our infant and early childhood experiences. In an ideal world the foundations would be adapted to the soil on which the building stands, being deeper and more extensive on lighter, less solid ground. In reality those early experiences are determined by many varied conditions and accidents of our birth and the temperaments of our parents.

Psychoanalytical theory and practice have revealed the importance of these earliest experiences in the shaping of our characters, and our sexuality must be seen as part of our total selves. However, this book is not about those early foundations, vital though they are. Those foundations are dealt with in the psychoanalytic literature and can only be explored by individuals through their relationship with a trained psychoanalyst or psychodynamic psychotherapist.

The concern of this book is the structure that is above the ground, that is, the more obvious building. We have to accept that the size and shape of the building, the personality, will be limited and affected by the given physical conditions and the man-made foundations. Yet the building that rises on those foundations is subject to tension, stresses and attacks at all stages of development.

The sexual life of the individual is particularly susceptible to such vicissitudes and may have become limited and inhibited within an otherwise fairly stable and well-developed personality. Thus a therapeutic approach of a more limited kind than that used by psychotherapists is possible. Main, in an article entitled 'Debt and Differentiation',[5] states that 'The psychosexual doctor learns to listen carefully, but is trying to hear a small, focused part of the unconscious material, in contrast to the psychoanalyst who must listen to everything.'

So far in this chapter I have suggested that there are some concepts that we can borrow from psychoanalysis and adapt for our purpose of using the relationship between the patient and the doctor in a therapeutic way. I am aware of the dangers of doing so, as to take the ideas and language of another discipline is to risk distorting the truths that have been explored within that other setting. I will return to the question of the importance of finding a suitable language for our work in the final part of this book. For now, there are a number of other ideas that we need to consider.

It is not easy for those of us who are not, as it were, working consciously with the unconscious to be able to imagine its realm. One of the most difficult things to believe is the existence of unconscious phantasy. We all know something of what Isca Salzberger-Wittenberg has called the 'top-layer' of phantasy,[10] that is, we know that we imagine and daydream. But the idea that there are primitive, often horrific, images in the deepest layers of the personalities of both children and adults is not an easy concept. However, if we can accept, albeit only on a rather intellectual level, that wild unconscious ideas and feelings do exist, we can move to a belief that such emotional matter could, in a sense, be forced out of oneself (projection) or taken in from others (introjection). Simple everyday examples abound. From my own experience I can remember the time when I furiously counted the piles of my husband's unsorted papers that littered the house, only to find when I stopped to count my own that there were even more. Or the time when, alone in my kitchen, I found myself saying *out loud* to myself, 'I really must tell my mother to stop talking to herself, people will think she is mad.'

When we begin to notice what we are feeling in a consultation it is possible to wonder whether some of that feeling has been pushed into us by the patient. How often is the doctor left feeling profoundly depressed, yet the patient seems to feel easier. 'Just listening' is not enough for any claim to a professional skill, but it is a beginning and may mean that we can help to contain some of the feeling for the patient.

Another word taken from psychoanalysis, and the last I want to consider in this chapter, is 'interpretation'. I have found myself going to the dictionary, where there are several suggestions for its definition: 'to explain the meaning of'; 'to translate into intelligible and familiar language'; 'to unfold, show the purport of'. I particularly liked the definition of an interpreter as 'one who translates between two parties', as I believe the body/mind doctor can translate between the two parties of the body and the mind.

The psychoanalyst might be thought of as translating the words of the conscious into the meaning of the unconscious. What sort of interpretation does the psychosexual doctor provide for his patient? Is it sensible to use the same word for something which must, by its very nature, be limited, both in the area of the personality being addressed and in the skill of the practising doctor? There is always a danger, as I have already mentioned, of using a word in everyday conversation and at the same time for a specific, technical purpose as part of a professional, theoretical structure. The difficulty is compounded when it is used by a number of allied disciplines, each giving it their own weight and nuances. Yet the idea that a doctor can use his observations of his own feelings and respond in such a way as to throw light on the dilemma of someone he is trying to help is a valid one.

We have seen that the psychosexual doctor, working with the body and mind together, has particular opportunities and responsibilities. The vulnerability of the physical examination exposes the patient to the possibility of making connections between bodily and emotional feelings. Time and again we hear our patients suddenly getting in touch with feelings they did not know they had. We might think of an interpretation in our field as a way of trying to help the patient make those connections.

When an interpretation is made it can be addressed to different levels of the personality. It has been suggested that in brief therapy the conscious ego should be addressed, although this will also speak metaphorically to the unconscious.[11] Certainly, the sort of remark designed to help the patient to feel you are on his or her side, including those interpretations based on the here-and-now feelings in the room, can make contact with less conscious levels. When a word or phrase echoes across the body/mind divide, it has particular power to penetrate some way into the depths of the psyche.[12] At these potent moments of body/mind doctoring it is almost as if the unconscious of the doctor speaks to the unconscious of the patient without going through the conscious of either of them. Something more than simple sharing of conscious feelings and explanation is taking place. In other words I believe we are in a position to make interpretations, albeit over a limited field of the personality of the patient.

Winnicott said, 'When I am working well I make two or three interpretations in a session. If I am tired this could be as many as six or seven, and when I am really exhausted I teach'.[13] How often we find ourselves teaching people about their bodies instead of wondering with them why they have not been able to find out for themselves from all the information available in the modern world.

In this chapter I have tried to relate some of the things that go on in a consulting room between patients and doctors to the theory and practice of psychodynamic workers. Such thinking does not mean that theoretical knowledge is necessary for whole-person doctoring. The work of doctors trained by the Institute of Psychosexual Medicine has shown that theory is not necessary, and it may even be a handicap to the development of skills to help patients. What is needed is the opportunity to practise working differently and to be able to discuss that practice with a group of colleagues in a structured way. Seminar training offers just that experience.

However, there is a recurrent call for theory, and I believe that the time may have come when we need to begin to think about how to describe our work more fully. I return to this subject in the final part of this book. For now, it is enough to say that I believe we have to look carefully at the language we use, adapting that used by other disciplines when it is suitable to the setting of general medical practice and body/mind doctoring. There is much we can learn from others, but we need to be selective and to subject any theory to the rigour of our own experiences in the consulting room with patients. Andrew Samuels, writing in another context, has said, 'It is the ethos, ideology, and method of the countertransference that should be shared with other disciplines, rather than models of the psyche, lists of defence mechanisms or schemas of personality development'.[14]

Those pioneers Michael Balint and Tom Main, in their work with generalist doctors, did not try to convert them to a psychoanalytic theoretical viewpoint. Instead they brought their deep understanding and experience of unconscious matters and put that at their disposal, remaining in ignorance about the work that was done in each particular setting. Such a shared ignorance mirrors the work that the doctor tries to do with the patient, a tolerance of not having the answer and not knowing what to do. It is the quality that is most likely to get lost when so called 'psychosexual experts' or even psychotherapeutic experts try to hand on their understanding. The ideas and insights in the following chapters are offered tentatively, in the hope that they will stimulate thought among doctors and others rather than being taken as some authoritarian view that could stifle the development of further work and ideas in this exciting field, where we are trying to understand aspects of the whole person.

References

1   Chesterton G K (1914) *The Defendant.* J M Dent, London.

2   James W (reprinted 1982) *The Varieties of Religious Experience.* Penguin, Harmondsworth.

3   Casement R (1985) *On Learning from the Patient.* Tavistock, London.

4   Main T (1989) Acquisition of Knowledge or Development of Skill? In *The Ailment and Other Psychoanalytic Essays* (ed. J Johns), Free Association Books, London.

5   Main T (1989) Debt and Differentiation. In *The Ailment and Other Psychoanalytic Essays* (ed. J Johns), Free Association Books, London.

6   Prospectus of the Institute of Psychosexual Medicine, available from 11 Chandos Street, Cavendish Square, London, W1M 9DE.

7   Lincoln R and Thexton R (1983) Retarded Ejaculation. In *The Practice of Psychosexual Medicine* (ed. K Draper), John Libbey, London.

8   Storr A (1979) *The Art of Psychotherapy.* Secker and Warburg, London.

9   Gill M (1989) Defences in the Doctor. In *Introduction to Psychosexual Medicine* (ed. R Skrine), Chapman & Hall, London.

10 Salzberger-Wittenberg I (1970) *Psychoanalytic Insights and Relationships.* Routledge, London.

11 Coren A (1996) Brief Therapy – Base Metal or Pure Gold? *Psychodynamic Counselling.* 2: 22–38.

12 Allen P, Wakley G, Skrine R and Smith A (1991) Deep Penetration on a Narrow Front. *Institute of Psychosexual Medicine Journal.* 2: 6.

13 Winnicott D W, quoted by Gosling R (1996). In *Michael Balint, Object Relations, Pure and Applied.* Routledge, London.

14 Samuels A (1993) *The Political Psyche.* Routledge, London.

Part II
Symptoms and Feelings

4

Making sense of symptoms

Physical and emotional pain is often easier to bear if one has an understanding of its cause, and both doctors and patients are anxious to find out why things happen. Even the act of giving something a name confines it, puts it in a category which is felt to be understood and which can be shared with others. Of course, there will be no sense of security, just the opposite if the category itself has uncontrollable or untreatable associations, as with 'cancer'. But for the worried mother of a fractious child a diagnosis of chicken pox or measles can bring relief, as she is now in the realm of the known.

I cannot be alone in having had the experience of feeling suddenly very unhappy, yet not being able to remember what triggered the feeling. When I can get in touch with the precipitating cause the mood lightens, as it does not then seem that the memory warrants such despair. Thus if we can remember, make connections with or even give names to some of the sources of our emotional pains, they become more manageable.

When we enter the field of sexuality, which is concerned with the body and mind acting together, the need to try to understand our feelings is very great, but diagnostic names are not very satisfactory. The name is better thought of as a symptom or sign, an outward complaint of an as yet undiagnosed state. The term 'sexual dysfunction' has been used to describe some of the common sexual difficulties, but to me the mechanistic overtones of such a phrase do nothing to help our understanding.

Some of the common sexual difficulties that are brought to doctors are listed in Table 4.1.

People who write about sexual difficulties use different and often idio-syncratic classifications of the problems they see, and I am no exception. For example, I have used the old-fashioned word 'frigidity' because I prefer it to 'non-orgasmic' or 'dysfunction of the arousal phase'. Frigidity describes something of the painful sense of being out of touch with feelings and also the atmosphere that can develop in the consultation, as described in the previous chapter. The doctor often becomes very active, as if chipping away

Table 4.1:   Classification of sexual symptoms

Women	Non-consummation
	Frigidity
	Dislike of any contact
	Sex tolerated but no arousal
	Arousal but no orgasm
	Lack of vaginal orgasm
	Dissatisfaction with orgasm
Men	Impotence
	Ejaculatory problems
	Too quick
	Unable to ejaculate
	Ejaculation with partial or no erection
Both	General lack of sexual interest in self or partner
	Anxieties about sexual matters, including gender, masturbation or unusual practices

at a block of ice with questions and ideas, yet somehow the patient, however hard she tries, cannot let out any feelings about the things that matter to her, except the despair of being how she is. One must, of course, identify what is meant by frigidity. Is it that awful feeling of not wanting even to be touched?: 'I am standing at the sink and he comes and puts his arms round me and I freeze.' What a terrible feeling. Is it that intercourse can be tolerated but in a totally passive way, almost as a martyr who 'lies there and thinks of England'. Often the complaint is of an inability to reach orgasm, even though she begins to get aroused and moist, before something creates a block and she turns off. In my experience such a woman often does not feel so cold in the consulting room, but she may block deeper exploration of her feelings.

Other complaints, such as lack of vaginal orgasm or dissatisfaction with the quality of the orgasms, also contain real sadness that has specific meaning for each individual.

In Table 4.1 I have listed the problems of men and women separately, but of course sex is an activity that takes place between two people. If the man has some degree of premature ejaculation (Kinsey *et al.* found in their survey that at least two-thirds of men would have liked to be able to last longer[1]), the woman may need to be very aroused before penetration if she has any hopes of reaching orgasm. I say 'may' because people are endlessly variable and I have known some women who can become orgasmic almost immediately following penetration with little foreplay.

As I write that paragraph I am aware at once of the limitation of such physical descriptions, as arousal and satisfaction for both partners, something which feels so easy and natural when it goes right and just happens, can be such a complicated process when things go wrong. In the following chapters I will explore further some of the feelings that can affect sexual activity, but here I am looking at the need to make sense of the symptoms that are presented and the difficulties that can arise for both those in trouble and those who try to help.

For many people the easiest path is to believe that the symptom has a purely physical cause. There may, of course, be some anatomical abnormality that, for example, can diminish the power of an erection in an older man. Such a physical waning of power is almost bound to be accompanied by feelings of anxiety, loss or anger, which in themselves may make the problem worse. The discomfort of admitting to feelings of any sort is a particularly British trait, the traditional 'stiff upper lip', and is not very helpful when trying to unravel the causes of sexual difficulties. For some, the denial of the emotional side of life leads the man to seek physical treatments in the form of penile injections or other devices, such as vacuum pumps. Such treatment can be helpful, both for those with substantial physical disease and for those who find that it can break the cycle of anxiety. Others find that such treatments have little effect or that the good results quickly wear off. In this situation they may find themselves wanting to explore other aspects of the problem. Other men who are more in touch with their feelings can sense that the blocks to their sexuality are likely to be in their minds. They may be able to have good erections when they masturbate, or with one woman but not another, demonstrating that their body can in some situations work normally.

The wish to find an understandable physical explanation for symptoms is equally strong in some women. For them, 'hormones' are often blamed. I believe that hormonal imbalance, certainly of a degree that can be shown by blood and other tests, is rare in women who have no other physical disease. Even at the menopause, hormone replacement therapy (HRT) may not restore a failing interest in sex. Although the improvement in the quality of the vaginal mucosa and the relief of dryness is appreciated by most women who take it, the time of the menopause is one at which many other changes are taking place in a woman's life. Children leave home, parents get older and need more care, there may be a chance to restart a career, or for those dedicated to a professional life there may be a dawning recognition that they have reached their peak. The situations are endless, and the specific meaning of the changes for each individual woman, both in relation to her feelings as a woman and to her relationship with her partner, where the balance between them may be disastrously altered, need to be explored. Very much against her conscious wish, such a woman may find she can no longer respond to her partner in the way she would like.

Another difficulty with diagnostic labels for sexual symptoms is one of definition. How can we, for example, define premature ejaculation? Caplan[2] points out that some people have tried to do so by reference to the length of time that vaginal containment can be enjoyed or the number of thrusts possible. Others have diagnosed it in terms of the partner's response: 'Long enough for the woman to reach orgasm on 50% of occasions'. What nonsense. How can one person's problem be defined in terms of another? Perhaps his partner has never been able to reach vaginal orgasm.

A number of men have never learnt to last very long, and anyone who could find some guaranteed simple cure for them could indeed become a millionaire. They may have tried the 'squeeze technique', first used by Masters and Johnson,[3] and I am sure that some people have found the method helpful, but I do not see them in my clinical work because people come to me when that method has failed and we have to try to explore the feelings together. When the squeeze technique does work I suspect that it does so by increasing the communication and reducing the tension between the couple, and thus the anxiety of the man, rather than by simple behavioural relearning.

Other men have gained good control but subsequently lose it under situations of psychic stress of various kinds. It is often not possible for such a man to understand the nature of the stress without help, as it usually arises from some change within himself or his relationship rather than from obvious worries about such things as work or money. Or to put it another way, what needs to be understood is the specific meaning of such external worries for the individual man, given that he is the person he is, with all his previous experiences, hopes, expectations and disappointments.

The first problem listed in Table 4.1, that of non-consummation, carries particularly poignant feelings for the couple. Usually, it is a very private difficulty, and it may have taken many years to be able to speak to anyone about it. Couples keep up a façade of normality. The woman may take the contraceptive pill regularly for many years, yet avoid any kind of physical examination at which there might be a chance for the problem to come to light. How often, when she goes for her repeat prescription of the pill, does she have to run for the bus, leave quickly because her boyfriend is waiting, or conveniently have a period, which in her eyes would be an absolute bar to examination? If examination does occur, she may give no clues that there is a problem and it can then be a disaster for her. One part of her is willing the doctor to solve the problem for her, while the other, very frightened part, is trying to protect her body. The procedure may well then be painful or even feel abusive, yet her sense of privacy and secrecy in that area of her body and feelings has made it impossible to protect herself by telling the doctor (or nurse) about the problem.

Perhaps of all the sexual difficulties brought to a body/mind doctor that of non-consummation is the one that demonstrates most clearly the wide diversity in type and seriousness of the underlying problems. Some couples can be easily helped by a gentle, sympathetic doctor who can explore with them their ideas about their bodies. Indeed, such exploration sometimes does not seem to be necessary, and simple support and reassurance appear to be enough. I am rather suspicious of these 'cures' as I believe that if there are still unrecognized phantasies about the body, confidence in its use will be fragile.

It is important to realize that both men and women can have what one patient called 'funny ideas' about their own and their partner's bodies. Because of these internal anxieties their sexual advances may be tentative, and they may often for this reason attract a partner who has fears of their own. Thus the inability to consummate the relationship becomes a collusive protection against anxiety.

Such personal body phantasies, which I will write about in more detail in a later chapter, are often best explored on a one-to-one basis with the doctor, but that does not mean that the partner may not need to be seen in his or her own right in a one-to-one situation, and sometimes work with the couple is also helpful. Some couples refuse to be separated, and the reasons for that need to be understood. Is it that one is defending the other from the phantasized attack of a brutal doctor? Or is there a fear that he or she will be attacked *in absentia* if the partner is left alone with the doctor? Do they imagine that they will be blamed if they are not there to defend themselves?

Many of those who cannot make love fully need time to mature within themselves as whole people. It is a clinical finding that many women who have been unable to allow penetration appear younger than their age and have difficulty breaking away from their parents. Such a generalization does not by any means always follow, as some have been extremely successful in their outside lives, seeming to have to compensate for an internal fear of being silly and cowardly, as they see it, by presenting a particularly efficient face to the world.

A powerful argument that couples can use to explain their sexual difficulties is that of moral or religious beliefs. There are, of course, even in today's society, people who choose to wait till they are engaged or married before they make love. While some may have taken such a decision from a position of genuine freedom, there are others who push their hidden, unacknowledged fears away behind a religious or intellectual shield. A blind faith that something which is not possible before marriage will somehow be 'all right on the night' is met by deep disappointment when they discover that the blocks are still present. In some ways the more genuine and sincere the belief, the more efficiently it acts as a defence. I have met couples who have clung to the belief that God will make it all right in his time, often for years after they are married, while the years of possible happiness and the prospects of fertility tick inexorably by.

For a few women and men the inability to have penetrative sex is part of a much deeper psychic problem. It has been suggested that non-consummation can be a defence against psychotic breakdown, so perhaps for those of us with painful memories of patients we have been unable to help there may be some consolation in knowing that we might have made them worse had we succeeded in removing their symptom. Such people are at the boundary of psychosexual work, and it is important for doctors to improve their diagnostic skills and liaise with those providing deeper and more long-term therapy if such patients are to be helped. I will return to the subject of non-consummation in the chapter on body phantasies, as it is an area in which body/mind doctors have much to offer.

It might appear from the word 'psychosexual' that problems such as anxieties about gender, or what are known as the perversions, such as trans-sexualism or transvestism, might fall within the remit of the body/mind doctor. (I am using the word 'perversions' here in a technical sense with no moral implications.) Such problems are thought to have their origins deep within the unconscious psyche, in an area referred to as the 'core complex'.[4] A few doctors working under the title 'psychosexual' have had extensive further training and are qualified to work in depth with such problems in a psychotherapeutic way, which is different from the brief approaches discussed in this book. For doctors trained only by the Institute of Psychosexual Medicine, such work is outside their competence. That is not to say that anxieties about such matters cannot be discussed, as doctors who are used to the everyday earthy matters of the body are less uncomfortable with the subject matter of unusual practices than are some other people. However, we would be charlatans if we believed or let our patients believe that what we have to offer can make a substantial difference to feelings that are very deep and often extremely distressing.

This is not the place, nor am I the person, to enter into a discussion of gender issues and the aetiology of lesbianism and homosexuality. Recent political action has forged a more comfortable place in society for such people, but there is still a long way to go before we can all be accepted for what we are. Psychoanalysis has produced theories of homosexuality,[5] but I suspect that the nature/nurture arguments are not over yet. From my own experience I am rather surprised at the comparatively small number of homosexuals or lesbians who come to ask for help with the ordinary problems of dysfunction and desire such as those being discussed in this book. Is this because they have fewer problems than heterosexual couples, or do they not feel entitled to ask for help? Perhaps the absence of children in most such relationships removes the need to stay together when sex goes wrong.

For those people who are in a muddle about their gender orientation, the body/mind doctor may be an appropriate person to talk to. One of the difficulties can be that hidden homosexual traits can confuse the doctor–patient relationship and may blind the doctor to sexual feelings developing within the consultation. I remember with shame two patients who had not acknowledged their hidden lesbian feelings (which I also had not recognized) who became overly attached to me. A properly trained psychodynamic psychotherapist offering more intensive therapy would probably have spotted what was happening and would have been able to understand it and use it as a transference phenomenon. I had to refer them for further help from more specialized therapists.

So far in this chapter I have been talking about direct requests for help with sexual problems. Many difficulties emerge during a consultation for some physical or emotional pain that may or may not have been connected in the patient's mind to sex. The sufferer may be aware of the true nature of the problem but be too shy to ask directly for help. This leads to what has been named the 'calling card', a physical problem being used in the hope that during the consultation there may be an opportunity to broach the more delicate subject. For other people there is no conscious recognition that there is an emotional or sexual content to their physical symptom. These are the people already mentioned in Chapter 2, who may be genuinely shocked to find themselves expressing feelings they did not know they had at the time of the physical examination.

The types of symptom that may be associated with a sexual difficulty are almost endless: contraceptive difficulties, genital and vague abnormal pains, menstrual upsets and a whole variety of anxieties and depressive feelings. Many of these complaints may have more than one cause, and doctor and patient have to try and untangle them together.

If we return to the efforts that people make to try and explain their sexual difficulties to themselves, we find that such explanations often confound and exacerbate the existing pain and difficulty.

Case Study 13

Mrs Lewis was a young woman who was referred to the psychosexual clinic without understanding what sort of doctor she was going to see. The problem was painful sex, and she said, 'I thought you were a psychiatrist, and that you would say I did not love my husband any more.' The doctor acknowledged the reality of the pain, and on examination managed to demonstrate that it was brought on by pelvic floor spasm. It was clear from the history that there had been a specific occasion when sex was painful, perhaps because at that time she had not been very interested or fully aroused, and she may have been a bit dry. One could surmise that she may not have felt particularly loving towards her husband at that moment, but that is quite a different matter from saying that she did not love him!

After that first shock of pain her body anticipated that it would be painful, and the spasm was the way in which her body tried to protect itself. For the body/mind doctor it was an easy matter to show her how she could control her muscles and bring the pain under control.

It was important to hear what Mrs Lewis said about not loving her husband, for despite her avowal and the doctor's belief that she did, there appeared to be some misunderstanding about the fact that love did not necessarily mean feeling loving at every minute of every day or night. The conflict that was present within her about the depth of her love was confused and made worse by her inability to understand the mechanics of her pain.

Our wish to find single explanations for our difficulties leads to a great deal of misunderstanding. One of the most painful experiences is to find that one's partner does not want, or cannot manage, to have sex. The immediate reaction is to blame oneself, or presume he or she has someone else. 'He has gone off me because I am too fat, not attractive enough...' is the thought of the woman who lacks confidence in her own attractiveness. Such may be the cause, but is seldom the simple answer that it sounds. Was there something unsatisfying in the relationship that made his eyes stray? Sometimes, especially after childbirth, the emotional experiences that the man has been exposed to have not been understood, and may have resonated with deeper fears and insecurities. The difficulty of seeing his woman as a wife and mother at the same time is one rather hackneyed example, but no less true for being obvious. The details of the experience and what it meant to that individual person need to be relived and understood.

It is often difficult for a woman to understand the sense of rejection that her man may feel if she does not want to make love. He will often accuse her of having a lover, yet she knows that is the last thing she wants. The loss is usually inside herself, and is concerned with losing touch with her own sexual feelings. How often have I listened to women saying 'I wouldn't mind if I never had it again with anyone.' Yet her partner feels it is a personal rejection of him. Neither of them can understand what is the cause of the problem, and indeed it is not easy to unravel.

Some of the feelings that can lie behind sexual problems are listed in Table 4.2. It is, of course, simplistic to list emotions in such a way, as they are not discrete entities at all. Grief can often contain much anger, anxiety is intimately tied up with shame and guilt, depression can increase feelings of vulnerability, and so on into an infinity of combinations. Again I provide a list just in order to try and define edges that can then be dissolved.

These feelings and some of the interactions between them will be explored in the following chapters. For now, I will return to the inadequacy, indeed the destructiveness, of the body/mind split within medicine and within individual people. The long tradition of keeping these two parts of ourselves separate makes it difficult to put them together at any level. It also provides an opportunity to project an internal emotional problem into the body and then onto the doctor whose task it is to care for the body. One woman spontaneously told me how frightening it was for her to consider the possibility that her mind could be causing her bodily symptoms. We take comfort in the belief that we are in control of our minds and that they would not do anything

Table 4.2:   Some emotions affecting sexual function

Fear of being 'that sort of girl' or boy
Fear of vulnerability and loss of control
Specific fear of body structures, e.g. a block
Specific fear of body function, e.g. wetness
Anxiety
Anger
Grief
Depression

so silly as to cause us pain. We badly need to believe that we are sensible and have difficulty forgiving ourselves for our desire to let go and, to some extent, to lose control. Yet to be sexual we have to be able to lose some control and, at its best, to get in touch with a 'silly' part of ourselves.

It is often easier to explain our problems in terms of someone else 'out there' who has done things to us, so that it is difficult to sort out what might be justifiable anger and resentment if experiences have indeed been painful. Such a feeling can be particularly strong following a bad experience of childbirth. At that time all one's sensory antennae are sharpened, and there is great vulnerability to a feeling of having been neglected or even attacked. Men and women who have not had an opportunity to come to terms with their experiences may have located the cause for their sexual difficulty in that experience and in the people whom they feel caused their suffering.

Case Study 14

Mrs Maggs complained that she had not had any desire for sex since the birth of her first child 13 years earlier. Her memories of the birth were still raw and vivid. It had been a difficult forceps delivery preceded by what had felt like a rough, uncaring and abusive vaginal examination. 'It felt like a rape', she said. The baby was in special care for several days, and Mrs Maggs felt excluded and not informed of his progress. Examination by the psychosexual doctor was surprisingly easy, and the vagina was found to be warm and relaxed. When the doctor commented on this Mrs Maggs said, 'Oh, I can always cut off and let them get on with it.' The doctor said perhaps that was the difficulty, she was too good at cutting off, and maybe that was what had happened to her feelings. This remark unleased a torrent of words about how her mother and grandmother had a horror of doctors, and of her father's death when she was a girl.

I cannot pretend that this short meeting produced any startling change in Mrs Maggs, but there was a softer atmosphere at her next visit and a wish to try to look at some other aspects of her life that might be playing a part in her problem. Having found the courage to face some strong feelings, she was able to begin to take a more realistic look at her experiences. It was possible for her to be less rigid in the way she explained her problem to herself, and therefore to entertain some hope of movement forward to a better state of affairs. For 13 years she had been stuck with one way of making sense of her predicament, putting the blame on those she felt had invaded her and robbed her of her privacy, but now there was a chance of looking at it, and feeling about it, differently.

One of the most unsettling states to be in is the inability to find any explanation for oneself. Some patients fall through the gap in the body/mind divide to such an extent that they can think they are going mad. I will finish this chapter with a simple but vivid example of how this can happen.

Case Study 15

Mrs Norris went to her general practitioner complaining of painful intercourse. He sent her to see a gynaecologist, who examined her and said there was nothing physically wrong. She was then sent to a psychiatrist, who said she was mentally normal. Within the confines of each medical specialty both views were reasonable. There was no anatomically fixed abnormality that was causing the pain, nor was there any sign of established mental illness. Mrs Norris, left with her pain, thought she was going mad. She felt they were both implying that she was imagining the pain, yet she knew it was real. She could find no method of explaining the pain to herself, became anxious and withdrawn and had to stop work.

It was not difficult for the psychosexual doctor to explain the body/mind interaction, the way in which she was unconsciously saying something with her body that she could not say in words. It emerged during the consultation that the content of this 'speech' was about her need to make love when she wanted to and not at the command of her husband. 'I want to give it as a gift when I want to', she said. Having voiced the feeling, she learnt to be able to do just that.

The effort to make sense of sexual symptoms can lead us all, patients and doctors alike, up many blind alleys. Patients need explanations for complicated happenings that cannot easily be explained. Doctors too want to have the power to provide such understanding. Yet the truth cannot be reached by striving to be clever, but only by staying in ignorance with the patient, working together in trust to try to understand. Then perhaps, as quoted on p. 3, some truth will 'emerge between two people looking for it'.[6]

References

1   Kinsey A C, Pomeroy W B and Martin C E (1948) *Sexual Behaviour in the Human Male*. W B Saunders, Philadelphia.

2   Caplan H C (1974) *The New Sex Therapy*. Baillière Tindall, London.

3   Masters W H and Johnson V E (1970) *Human Sexual Inadequacy*. J and A Churchill, London.

4   Glasser M (1992) The Management of the Perversions, with Special Reference to Transvestism. In *Psychosexual Medicine* (ed. R Lincoln), Chapman & Hall, London.

5   Lewes K (1989) *The Psychoanalytic Theory of Male Homosexuality*. Meridian, New York.

6   Symington N (1986) *The Analytic Experience*. Free Association Books, London.

'I'm not that sort of girl' – or boy

I have taken my title for this chapter from a story told by a visiting American sexologist many years ago. He was working with a group of young pregnant girls, who sat in a circle with the evidence that they had been sexual plainly visible for all to see. One of the main concerns they all wished to talk about was the fact that they were not 'that sort of girl'. They were anxious not to be thought promiscuous, loose or whorish, and to persuade themselves and each other that their pregnancies were the result of love rather than of unbridled sexual passion.

Nowadays some of the unconscious reasons for early pregnancy are better understood: they are concerned with the sense of being unloved or unlovable, and the need to have something of one's own to love. Many women who embark on sexual adventures very early in their lives get little physical pleasure for themselves. Their love affairs are usually part of an effort to find independence from their parents, and the emotional involvement with their partner becomes a pale shadow compared with the loves and hates felt within their own nuclear family. Deeper conflicts can be reawakened as they use this time of emotional turmoil to work through some of the unresolved conflicts belonging to the past.[1]

This chapter is not concerned primarily with adolescence, but with the sense of not wanting to be 'that sort of girl' that can be felt at all ages. As doctors who are used to talking about the details of the workings of the body, we can sometimes see how closely the sense of anxiety and disgust is linked to the sensations of physical arousal. It is tempting to think mainly of women in this chapter, but parallel difficulties can be present in men and I will include them when I can. The internal anxieties about 'What sort of man am I?', which may or may not have been settled to some degree during adolescence, can be reawakened at various times during a man's life in the same way as can anxieties about what it means to be a woman. Sexual confidence may have become established, only to be rocked by the various life changes to which we are all heirs. The strain of long-term relationships, pregnancy and childbirth, or the absence of children for whatever reason, middle age, the menopause and old age have somehow to be negotiated. Outside events such as unemployment or illness can unsettle and disintegrate the picture of oneself as a whole man or woman, able to be at the same time loving and sexual, silly and responsible, grown-up and childish.

As I search for examples from my own work and that of my colleagues, I feel almost overwhelmed by the diversity and depths from which I am trying to pluck a few real moments when a doctor and patient have together understood something in such a way that a block has been released and freedom found. Samuels warns of the need to be wary of case examples as they can be grossly manipulative.[2] One remembers the moments when light suddenly shone in, and forgets the darkness and lack of understanding that went before and may well, for all we know, have followed afterwards. Brief clinical encounters may be skewed in the memory, and we must be careful not to make extravagant claims. I hope that the image of the doctor, not as an all powerful, active agent, but as a facilitating catalyst whose role is to help the patient make his own connections, will do something to offset any aura of omnipotence that these case vignettes may give.

The following example describes a particularly explicit memory that was blocking the way to full sexual expression and that was recaptured during brief psychosexual therapy.

Case Study 16

Mrs Osborne was a married woman in her mid-30s with three children. She was referred because she had never been able to have an orgasm and this was causing strains in the marriage. She told the doctor that she loved her husband very much but that her inability to respond to him as she and he both wanted was a source of great conflict and sadness. They had faced considerable difficulties within the family as they had a handicapped child, and in addition the husband was not always able to find work. In order to supplement their income she had to work, so was often very tired.

As the story unfolded, the doctor felt there could be many obvious reasons why she might not want to make love. Anxiety about the children, overtiredness and financial worries all appeared to be at the forefront of her mind and dominated the conversation during the first consultation. The doctor was tempted to reassure her and explain that such pressures frequently interfered with love-making, but, remembering that the complaint was of *never* having had an orgasm, she managed to keep quiet.

At their second meeting the patient appeared quieter and more thoughtful. After a relaxed and easy vaginal examination Mrs Osborne began to talk about her adolescence. Her father had been very strict and she had to be in the house each night at 9 pm. If she was as much as 5 minutes late, he would put his head out of the window and shout, 'You slut, you whore.' She felt that all the street could hear him. The irony was that she had never ever had sex before she married, and in fact had allowed nothing more than some kissing and fondling above the waist. Now she could admit that she did enjoy love-making and would begin to get aroused, but then she would remember her father's voice and turn off, preventing herself from reaching any sort of enjoyable orgasm.

For this patient the memory of that humiliation was so painful that she had suppressed it, and it was only in the presence of a doctor who was interested in sexual feelings, and perhaps as a result of surviving a vaginal examination without too much embarrassment, that she had been able to allow herself to remember it again. Once she had done so it did not take her long to give herself permission to enjoy her body.

Most people are not subjected to such obvious and explicit denigration of their sexuality: the prohibitions that they have built into themselves are more subtle. I am frequently surprised at how little attention is paid to these internal blocks to the enjoyment of sex in sex manuals. Instructions in sexual technique, and suggestions about different positions and activities to heighten pleasure and excitement seem irrelevant to many of the people I meet. As one woman said, 'I only want to be able to do it in bed in the ordinary way.' A woman who has found her way to orgasm may be very put off by suggestions that she should be able to enjoy more imaginative and varied activity. What may seem to her partner as prudishness or lack of initiative may be her fear that change will put her off. She may be very aware of the fragility of her own arousal.

Inhibition of sexual response can happen at any time and can be particularly baffling when it happens out of the blue in what has until then been a mutually satisfying and exciting relationship. I am fearful for the woman who says she must be sure that sex is all right before she commits herself to a relationship by getting engaged or married, as it is often at that time that things can go wrong.

Case Study 17

Mrs Pearce went to the doctor complaining of sudden and complete loss of interest in sex. She described vividly how she knew the exact moment when it happened. She was walking through a park on a lovely spring day 6 weeks after her marriage. The trees were in blossom and the birds were singing, but she suddenly thought to herself, 'I have caught my man, I never have to do it again.' From that moment she could not let her husband near her.

For some time the doctor too could not get near her. The consultation felt cold, clinical and sensible. The doctor became active, prodding and full of good ideas. Slowly, it dawned on her that the awful frigidity inside this patient was being projected into the room and into herself. She had to tolerate the unyielding atmosphere of common sense and control, until after several sessions the patient was able to start to talk about her home life.

She had been brought up in a house full of women. Her mother, aunt and grandmother lived together, and the prevailing belief was that men only wanted 'one thing'. There was a patronizing view of men as little boys who had to be humoured and looked after, and that if you were to catch them and keep them you had to submit to sex from time to time. The idea that there could be anything pleasurable for the woman was implicitly denied.

Despite this background Mrs Pearce had very much enjoyed her sex life at the beginning. While 'catching her man' she had been able to let herself go, and there had been much pleasure in flouting the accepted, unstated view that such behaviour was not acceptable in 'nice women'. Once she herself became that respectable thing, a married woman, she lost touch with the other side of herself. It took her some time to mature enough to make her own decisions about what sort of woman she wanted to be, and to break away from the role models she had been presented with while she was growing up.

For women such as Mrs Osborne and Mrs Pearce it is seldom enough for their doctor to try to give them permission to enjoy their sexual lives. Encouragement to 'come on in, the water's lovely' can feel like a real denial of the internal problem and makes the patient feel misunderstood. The degree to which such encouragement is felt as inappropriate can be sensed in the doctor, who is made to feel too sexy and 'not quite nice' herself. The woman has to learn to give herself permission and needs the help of a doctor who can work with her to understand the blocks. She will often blame her parents for being so inhibiting, yet not everyone who sees their parents as overly strict has problems. Exchanging a mental image of a restricting, inhibiting parent for an allowing, encouraging doctor does little good. Finding someone who can stay with them while they think about the meaning of the half-felt, half-understood emotions is quite a different matter.

How can we begin to understand the strength of these inhibiting feelings? It seems to me that it is more a matter of shame than of guilt. I have been pondering the difference as I think about these women. All the definitions of shame that I can find in the dictionaries contain overtones of exposure: 'a humiliating feeling of having appeared to disadvantage in one's own eyes or those of others ... fear of incurring disgrace or dishonour'. Guilt, on the other hand, is defined as a state of having done wrong: sin ... sinfulness ... having broken the law. Dr Michael Conran[3] has said that shame is the poison of thought and feeling, and that embarrassment is a form of benign shame. On the other hand, one needs to be able to think in order to feel guilty.

What then is this shame about the fact of bodily sexual arousal? I suspect that it goes back to our earliest experiences and is connected with the unconscious fantasies that were associated with those infantile and childish sexual feelings. Here I am getting out of the realm of ordinary body/mind doctoring and into depth psychology, and I do not wish to suggest that it is necessary to go that far in order to help many of those who choose to come to us. Symington says that 'Shame is the emotion we experience when we are aware of the parts of ourselves that are not integrated'.[4] The fear, the need to hide that part of ourselves that we do not like, be it felt in our bodies or as part of our emotions, is confronted by the exposure and inevitable vulnerability that is present during a physical examination.

Let me take you back to Miss Evans on p. 19. You may remember that she was unable to have an orgasm and, during a routine check of her vaginal diaphragm, she was able to say that she was afraid of being silly and making a noise if she let herself go. What seemed particularly important for her was that the doctor continued to see her as a sensible, reasonable person, a view she was afraid her parents did not have of her. In this way the doctor was able to hold and value both sides of her, so that she had a momentary experience of having those two parts of herself integrated within one person, and was then able to integrate them within herself.

Every physical examination has the potential for embarrassment, which we have seen can be considered as a benign form of shame. If the inevitable exposure and vulnerability can be survived by the patient without it making her feel destroyed, she may then feel safe enough to allow further emotions and memories to surface. Some of the roots of the shame may then be brought to consciousness, where they can be more easily dealt with. Such I believe is what happened with Mrs Osborne above, who after a vaginal examination, was able to share her painful memories of her father's scorn.

Of course, we cannot totally separate shame and guilt, and both can be aroused by many different outside events. A woman may have managed to make enough contact with the grown-up independent person inside herself to develop a satisfactory sexual life, but such contact may be fragile and easily lost. Any disease or disorder of the genital part of herself is particularly likely to push such a vulnerable person into a state of despair and disgust at her own body and its arousal. Independence, both in practical living and in sexual expression, may be hard-won.

Case Study 18

Miss Quinn was an only child of elderly devoted parents. It was not until she was 30 years old that she managed to live away from home in her own flat and find a boyfriend. Their sexual life began to develop and she was beginning to enjoy it, but on routine screening she was found to have an abnormal smear. This was a disaster for her. She felt that it was punishment for her sexual interest and was unable to continue to make love. Her sense of guilt and shame was such that she was not able to have any real contact with a psychosexual doctor, and within 4 months she had sold her flat and was again living at home with her parents.

The epidemiological evidence that cancer and precancer of the cervix is in some way associated with sperm makes every woman who has an abnormal smear potentially at risk. It needs someone who is very confident in her sexuality to survive the unspoken or imagined comment or even censure of her sex life to win through unscathed. Genital infections can act in the same way. One woman was unlucky enough to develop genital herpes after the second occasion on which she ever made love. She went on to marry the man involved, but was still having painful sex with no enjoyment 2 years later. Her anger was great, and it seemed as if she needed to hold on to her pain in order to prove to her mother, her husband and her doctor that 'a nice girl like me should not have got a dirty disease'.

For men too the advent of a sexually transmitted disease can be devastating. Feelings of guilt about an illicit relationship can be so great that a persecutory fear of AIDS can develop. The feeling that 'I have been so bad that I deserve to die' can lead a man to travel from clinic to clinic asking for repeated tests. Such a phobia may have taken over where there was already a fragile integration of the 'dirty' sexy side of themselves with their loving feelings, and all further sexual responses may be inhibited. What seems to be an overt, conscious guilt that can be thought about and acknowledged is complicated by a deeper sense of shame that may sabotage any reparative wishes by making him impotent with the woman he loves.

Shame, guilt and anger are so inextricably mixed that it is often difficult to do more than contain whichever is being expressed at the moment, while trying to remain open to the underlying complicating feelings. Other illnesses, such as malignancies, in men and women can evoke many of the same feelings. Listening to a psychoanalyst talking about the impact of gynaecological cancer,[5] I felt very much at home. Here were the same feelings of guilt about such previous sexual activities as masturbation, abortion and frequent sexual partners, and shame, which she defined as a specific form of anxiety evoked by the imminent danger of unexpected exposure, humiliation or rejection.

It may seem strange that I have got this far in the book without saying much about childhood sexual abuse. It is not because we do not see adults who have been abused as children in psychosexual medicine. Indeed, about 10% of psychosexual patients give a history of some such occurrence.[6,7] However, we are seeing a select group of people who have chosen to come to a doctor for help with sexual problems rather than with more general personality problems or mental illness. Many of our abused patients do not seem to stand out as being very different from other people when they are trying to make sense of their sexual difficulties. General remarks about the importance of sexual abuse in the aetiology of later sexual difficulties must be seen as relating to the particular group of people being studied, and as such a psychosexual clinic population provides a useful research cohort,[8] provided one takes account of the setting in which they present their problem.

The most striking clinical impression of patients who give a history of sexual abuse is the wide difference in degree of damage that has been done. For some the whole personality seems to have been shattered, and one cannot imagine a future that will not require much long-term support and practical help. For many others the abuse, which may be presented as an important memory, quickly becomes irrelevant. In today's society it may be easier to explain one's problem in terms of abuse rather than struggling to understand more complicated feelings within oneself or within a relationship. Indeed, much is now described as abuse that would previously have passed for an unfortunate experience, such as genital exposure or body contact in public places. The impact on the individual person is what matters.

It seems appropriate to consider sexual abuse in this chapter, as the legacy is so often one of guilt for not stopping it or even for the belief that he or she encouraged or asked for it. Shame too can be intense, especially if there was physical response or pleasure. As Wakley says, 'It is impossible to be stimulated sexually without responding in some way'.[9] The memory of physical arousal under what are felt to be secret and often sinful conditions can become embedded in the adult and then contributes to the sense of being a wickedly oversexed person. It is not surprising that such a fear can lead to the unconscious control of sexual arousal. Such control will often present as a complaint of frigidity, as the fear is well hidden. At the other extreme sexual feelings may be denigrated as part of a sense of general worthlessness, and promiscuous but usually joyless sex can result.

The fear of finding a ravening sexual beast inside is by no means only confined to those who have been sexually abused. It can be difficult to suggest to a profoundly frigid woman that such might be the case, and the doctor can only hold the idea at the back of his or her mind so that clues dropped by the patient can be heard. Suggestions along such lines will fall on stony ground if they are produced as good ideas rather than as a response to something picked up from the patient herself.

When I try to consider further the boy or man who has difficulty putting the different parts of his sexuality together, the loving, the aggressive, the dirty, I feel I am on less solid ground. Is this because I am not a man and cannot use my own experiences to reverberate with his? I think it is more likely to be lack of clinical experience in this area. Psychosexual medicine grew out of family planning, and I and my colleagues of the same generation started by seeing more women than men. We now see far more men, and we are learning, but I feel less confident about forecasting which patients may be helped by a brief psychosexual approach and which will need more extensive therapy.

Certainly, I have seen a number of men who have difficulty putting the image of the 'Madonna' with that of the 'whore'. They can be effectively sexual with women they do not care about and whom they can allow to be sexual beings, but woe betide them when they really fall in love. I suspect that this split can be found in every degree from the fairly mild to the deep and serious. I have certainly seen a few men for whom I could do nothing, despite my best attempts to be felt as a woman who was respectable, a mother, but also a sexual being interested in sexual things. Other men may be helped, using the same techniques of the doctor–patient relationship and the physical examination. Mr Holden, described briefly on p. 22, was someone who was relieved to be able to talk about his confusion regarding sex with nice women, after surviving the anxiety about whether or not he was expected to have an erection during the examination.

Sometimes the split between the woman with whom he can be sexual and the 'pure' Madonna image only occurs after they have had a baby. Such a reaction can be devastating for both people. So often the woman feels he has gone off her because she is no longer attractive following the physical changes of pregnancy, and the man can make no sense of his feelings. It is, as always, important to try to look at the details of the experience for the individual.

Other changes in the family can also produce sexual difficulties but the connections may be less obvious.

Case Study 19

Mr Daniels asked for help because of impotence for the last 2 years. He was a middle-aged man who enjoyed his beer on a Saturday night with the lads. He had sustained a loving and happy relationship with his wife until he became impotent, but now he wondered whether he should follow the example of some of his mates and see if it would work with someone else.

As he talked to the doctor, the answer to the question 'Why then?' became a bit clearer. At about the time he became impotent his daughter was found to be taking drugs. He was very upset, but it was not until the third visit, following a physical examination, that he began to talk about an episode when his daughter was 11 years old. He had been teaching her to swim at the local pool and had inadvertently touched her developing breast. Whether or not that had been exciting for him was not discussed and perhaps did not need to be. His horror that it might have been was enough to make him withdraw from further swimming lessons and indeed from physical contact of any sort with his daughter.

It is interesting that he did not become impotent at that time, but only at the time when he found out his daughter was taking drugs several years later. It was then that the fear that he might have seriously damaged her by his clumsiness, his sexiness or even his withdrawal made him suppress all sexual feeling within himself. Discussing such fears with a doctor who was not shocked or damaged by them, but who could interpret his fear that his

feelings might be damaging to one he loved, was enough for him
to allow himself to feel sexual towards his wife again.

In this case it could have been tempting to rush in and interpret the
impotence in general terms relating to anxiety about his daughter or the
stresses her problems might have caused in his relationship with his wife. Such
haste would have denied the possibility of getting in touch with the more
personal, painful and potent hidden feeling that lay behind his impotence.

Many questions remain unanswered about this man. For example, we
know nothing about the type of personality he was at a deeper level or what
had predisposed him to be so sensitive to the fear that his sexual feelings
might be inappropriately displaced. Such knowledge would require long-term
therapy that he was not asking for and was unlikely to welcome, even if it had
been available. A brief body/mind approach had allowed him to make some
connections that restored his manhood.

There are many situations in later life when sexual interest or response
may become inhibited. The burgeoning sexuality of children can be threatening to their parents. It has been suggested that it is difficult for daughters to
be sexually happy if they feel their mothers are not, but in a reciprocal way
there are parents whose own sex lives may be stunted if they are anxious
about those of their children. The fervent hope that their child is 'not that
kind of girl' arouses fears and perhaps shame about the rectitude of their own
arousal. Practical fears about pregnancy and infections are infused by wider
anxieties and moral concerns, and social and historical attitudes to sexuality
lying buried within the individual are hard to change.

Case Study 20

Mrs Rice went to the doctor in deep distress about her loss of
sexual interest within a happy marriage. She had negotiated
the menopause successfully, and continued to have a fulfilling,
although less frequent, sexual life with her much loved husband.
She could not understand why she had suddenly, 1 year previously, found that her body no longer responded. HRT had made
the act more comfortable but had done nothing to restore her
feelings.

It was not until her second meeting with the doctor, who
was puzzling about what else had been going on in her life at
the time of the change, that she was able to say that they had
discovered that their son was homosexual. Both she and her

husband considered themselves to be liberal and understanding. They had welcomed his partner and believed that they had come to terms with the situation. Only in the privacy of their own bedroom, far from the needs of political correctness and her deeply held wish to accept all aspects of her son, did her body, against her conscious wishes, express her innermost feelings.

Thus to old age, and the hope that despite failing physical powers, the closeness and warmth of body contact can be maintained. Gilley,[10] using the term 'sexuality' in its broadest sense, defines it as 'the capacity of the individual to link emotional needs and physical intimacy – the ability to give and receive physical intimacy at all levels, from the simplest to the most profound'. It is here that earlier inhibitions, for example about touching and non-penetrative sex, can limit the options for closeness, although Gilley puts this in the wider setting of the total personality in her moving and illuminating remarks about terminal care.

The depth to which sexual expression, when it is not inhibited by shame, reaches into our feelings and releases them was shown to me when I was working in general practice. An old man, who had suffered repeated strokes, was dying at home. One day as I sat with his wife, she wept and told me how, the night before when she had 'You know doctor, tried to help him with my hand', he had rejected her. Despite his long illness it was the first time in their life together that such a thing had happened, and for her it was the moment of parting. When he died 2 days later she was dry-eyed and practical. The rupture caused by the end of intimacy had broken through the protective shell of this courageous woman so that I could, just for a moment, share her grief. I felt privileged to do so.

References

1 Pines D (1993) *A Woman's Unconscious Use of her Body: A psychoanalytical perspective*. Virago Press, London.

2 Samuels A (1989) *The Plural Psyche*. Routledge, London.

3 Conran M (1995), quoted at an open meeting at the Institute of Psychoanalysis, London.

4 Symington N (1993) *Narcissism: A new theory*. H Karnac, London.

5   Springer-Kremser M (1992) Psychosocial and Sexual Impact of Gynaeco-
    logical Cancer. In *Reproductive Life: Proceedings of the 10th Interna-
    tional Congress on Psychosomatic Obstetrics and Gynaecology* (eds. K
    Wijma and B von Schoultz), Parthenon Publishing, Carnforth.

6   Morgan A (1990) A Study of Patients with a History of Sexual Abuse.
    In *Proceedings of the Fifteenth Scientific Meeting of the Institute of
    Psychosexual Medicine*, IPM, London.

7   Skrine R (1991) Audit of a Psychosexual Clinic: Pattern of attendance
    and outcome, Great Britain. *Journal of Public Health Medicine*. 13: 3.

8   Van Hegan G, Tunnadine P, Kwantes E. *Treatment of Psychosexual
    Disorders in Previously Abused patients*. In press.

9   Wakley G (1991) *Sexual Abuse and the Primary Care Doctor*. Chapman
    & Hall, London.

10 Gilley J (1992) Intimacy and Terminal Care. In *Psychosexual Medicine*
    (ed. R Lincoln), Chapman & Hall, London.

6

Body fantasies

The idea of using the word 'block' in the title of this book came to me as I thought about all the patients who talk about a block. It may be located in the vagina ('Nothing can get in, I feel there is a block'), in the penis ('Something is blocking me from ejaculating') or in the emotions. I am still repeatedly surprised by the detail and individual differences in the mental images of the bodily block and the way in which one fantasy, once it has been explored, can be replaced by another and then another.

What is the relation between these 'funny ideas' that people have about their bodies and the sense of themselves as whole people? Where do the ideas come from? Working in a body/mind way, we can sometimes begin to find an answer to the first of those questions, but the second one is much more difficult. I have previously mentioned the need that we have to make sense of our pains, and one of the most pressing questions that may be asked, for example by a woman unable to consummate her marriage, is 'Why am I like this?'

In the present climate there is often an assumption that it has been caused by childhood sexual abuse. Such may be the case, but in my experience that is unusual. Indeed, much anguish can be caused by searching for evidence of abuse. My suspicion is that some people are susceptible to muddle about their personal anatomy and physiology from very early times in their life. Misunderstandings about the physical differences between men and women, confusions about what holes there are, and which things go into and come out of each, may put the individual at risk of confusion that can be made worse by later events. For example, one patient with multiple body fantasies vividly remembered the occasion when a girl at school fell on a bamboo and damaged herself somewhere 'down below'. She had had to go to hospital, and there had been some bleeding, but the exact nature of the damage remained a mystery, which was made worse by the secrecy both at school and at home. The experience did nothing to help her clarify what I am sure were pre-existing muddles about the holes and where they were.

We may have to accept that we will not be able completely to understand the genesis of body fantasies. It is likely that we all have misunderstandings about our bodies at a deeply unconscious level. Yet the majority of people overcome such blocks during the process of psychological development and find their way to using their bodies reasonably well to express their sexuality. However, our lack of full understanding does not detract from our ability to help many, although not all, patients to get in touch with their unconscious ideas and images of their own and their partners' bodies. Indeed, someone who can work with the body and mind together may be the best person to offer such help, as many other therapists are barred from direct access to the body. Standing by a couch where a patient is lying or sitting within the privacy of a surrounding curtain, it may be possible to give confidence that a finger, the doctor's or the patient's, could be allowed to slip in without causing damage. Such self-exploration may be accompanied by delighted surprise and possibly excitement. Sometimes the self-exploration itself can be therapeutic, but if either doctor or patient expects it to work a sort of magic, they are laying themselves open to intense disappointment. It is essential that the patient's disappointment is openly acknowledged, and that the doctor can recognize his or her own, so that both can find a renewed energy and hopefulness to tackle the difficult problem of exploring the fantasies.

How is this done? At this point I find myself in a dilemma. How helpful would it be to share some of the many detailed fantasies that I and my colleagues have come across in our work? I am tempted to reproduce some of the drawings that patients have made in their search to explain their ideas, as they are vivid and extraordinary. But everyone is different, and perhaps it is just because of this individuality that I have decided not to show them. A visual picture could become too powerful in the mind, and a patient or doctor might try to force the image that is emerging between them into one shown here. Yet the more experienced doctor does have the advantage of knowing something of the similarities as well as the individual differences and can formulate a range of general possibilities at the back of his or her mind. It is against this background knowledge that the doctor has to listen acutely, with all the senses, to the faint clues that the patient may give about her inner pictures of her body. It is important to stress that the patient is not aware of these images until the doctor helps her to find them; she is truly unconscious of them.

Is it fanciful to suggest that at this moment there is something of a parallel with the work of the psychoanalyst who, with many theories at the back of his mind, strives in any particular session to wait in the presence of the patient, with 'evenly suspended attention'?[1] Of course, as Main has pointed out, we do not have to listen to everything.[2] Our focus, especially at the moment of physical examination, is on the patient's body image, and in particular the image of the genitals and associated structures, and the ideas of how they work.

Even within the limitations of our field of interest there is another difference from the psychoanalytic world, in that we do not have well-developed theories of psychosexual medicine to hold at the back of our minds. Such theories can only grow out of the study of clinical work, and I will return to the need for and the difficulties of formulating such theories in the final part of this book. For now, I will try to give a preliminary framework of the general nature of body fantasies as I have found them in the patients whom I have seen. Such a structure will need to be modified and developed in the light of further experience.

Table 6.1 lists some of the ideas about the vagina that patients have shared with me. Fantasies about the penis will be dealt with later. Most of the ones listed have come from women unable to consummate their relationships, although the dangerous nature of the vagina, especially the sense that it contains teeth, is more commonly expressed by men. It is not difficult to see how that can be an expression of how he may feel unconsciously about one side of the whole woman.

In Table 6.1 I have not included those fantasies that can emerge later, for example after childbirth or at the menopause. The idea of having been stitched up wrongly is now well known, although eliciting this fantasy (if it is a fantasy) may not be easy. The sense of having been damaged by the baby, or by the medical attendants, can become fixed in the vagina or on the perineum and will be discussed further in Chapter 8.

The listing of mental images in the way I have done in the table is a crude way of organizing the clinical material that is such a private part of a person's self. It tells us neither anything of what the mental image means for the patient as a whole person, nor of the atmosphere between the doctor and patient as the fantasy was discovered between them. Yet I have felt it important to try to emphasize the detail of the exploration that is needed by some patients if they are going to be able to overcome the fear that produces vaginismus.

In women who cannot consummate their relationships the most usual fear is of pain, perhaps accompanied by damage and bleeding. I wonder how much of this we can lay at the door of the 'bodice-ripper' novels. Such books have arisen from within our culture and must be expressing deeply held myths about the hymen, the 'maidenhead', the state of virginity and its loss. Certainly, the unrealistic idea that the penis will enter the first time with searing pain, bleeding, and at the same time deep and earth-moving pleasure, is still present in many of these patients. Men too, often the partners of such women,

Table 6.1:   Vaginal fantasies

The entrance	Blocked
	    Partially
	    Completely
	Hidden
	Absent
	Within another entrance (cloacal)

The passage	Very small Blocked Curved Absent – has to be made by breaking Dangerous – e.g. with teeth Disgusting – e.g. slimy, 'ugh'
The wall	Rigid Fragile – 'like tissue paper' Corrugated – easy to lose one's way Raw – 'like raw meat'
The top	Joins directly to the womb Frightening cavity – 'things can get lost' Leads into insides – 'he might touch my liver'

may have fears of the damage and pain they will have to cause, perhaps hiding deeper fears that such aggression might be enjoyable.

When working with such patients I am usually the one who first uses the world 'hymen', and sometimes it is difficult to do so. It is as if the very use of the word is a sort of rape. Once the word is in the open, lying in the space between doctor and patient, it may be possible to explore what it means to the patient. Often it is imagined as a membrane right across. When asked how the menstrual blood gets through the reply is 'It oozes through' or 'By a sort of osmosis'. The relief, and sometimes the disappointment, when the tip of the doctor's finger is eased past can be intense. Other patients, while appearing to believe that the hymen has been passed, cannot give up the fantasy so easily. In their minds the drum-like membrane can seem to move up the vagina in front of the advancing finger, either her own or the doctor's, and come to cover the cervix. Here the image may get muddled with ideas about the need to 'break through into the womb'.

Some women have a fairly realistic idea of the structure of the hymen, although they seldom see it as something that is made to stretch easily. Others think it is thick, perhaps extending to a depth of an inch or two and needing to be torn throughout its thickness. Can we wonder at their fear?

Many women without these problems will have explored their vagina as an infant or small child as a part of pleasurable masturbatory activity, and then again at adolescence, often when wanting to use internal tampons. The inability to insert a tampon may be the first conscious awareness that there is a problem, but it is often pushed away with the thought that it will be 'all right when I fall in love', 'all right when we are married', 'all right when it is right with God'.

It may come as a surprise that many couples who cannot consummate their relationship can still have an enjoyable love life with mutual masturbation. The fears in these women, and often the men they have chosen, are usually very specifically about penetration. The hymen can perhaps be considered as one of the guardians of the entrance, but for some women the labia, or lips, are another. I remember one woman saying, as I parted the labia before inserting a finger, 'There is an outer and inner part of me, the curtains have to be drawn.' Anxieties about the unequal size of the labia were mentioned on p. 11 when I discussed the need to relate the anxiety to fear of damage by masturbation. I have met several women who felt deformed by what they felt to be the excessive size of their labia, one remembering a time when she was in the bath with several other little girls who mocked the way that part of her body looked. The saddest of these women are those with very normal and often beautiful bodies, who nevertheless want their labia, or their breasts reduced or 'tidied up'. Brief psychosexual therapy is unlikely to change their minds or to deflect them from such self-mutilation.

I used to believe that cloacal fantasies could be laid at the door of biology teachers who used animals as their subjects rather than humans. Now I think that they were perhaps only expressing a more general unconscious muddle about the holes and where they are. Nevertheless, it is still not uncommon to find beautiful drawings of the ovaries, fallopian tubes and uterus, and even of the perineum, but the part between is often small and not clear. Is this a cultural expression of the fact that the little girl cannot see her vagina, whereas the little boy has the reassurance of seeing his penis? McDougall points out that 'Since her sex is, in essence, a portal into her body, the vagina is destined to be equated in the unconscious with anus, mouth and urethra'.[3] Certainly, I have often voiced a patient's complaint that God was not very clever when he put what should be a pleasurable hole so near to those that can be associated with dirt and disgust in the adult. We must remember, however, that the anus is a place that gives much pleasure to the infant. This pleasure is in part the sensory feeling of the contraction of smooth muscle in the action of defecation and may also have provided comforting masturbatory sensations. The anus and its function also become associated with the pleasure of giving and withholding gifts.

Returning to the question of what such ideas about the body might mean in terms of the whole person, we have to look to the relationship between the doctor and patient for evidence. On p. 33 I wrote about a patient who was so controlling that the doctor drove her home and wrote notes in her diary about not being late. I do not think we can explain this need to control those around her as well as her own body only in terms of the fear of the physical pain of penetration, strong though that was. It is worth considering whether there was also a threat to her sense of the integrity of her whole being.

Joyce McDougall, working as a psychoanalyst with patients over a long period of time, has looked at some of those illnesses that are thought to have psychosomatic causes lying deeply within the personality and originating early in infancy and childhood. One such illness is eczema and she postulates that it is a response to anxieties about the boundaries of the self.[4] As a body/mind doctor I have to consider that idea as but one factor among many possible aetiological causes of eczema, including genetic inheritance and immunological frailties. Nevertheless, the subsidence of a variety of symptoms in her patients following prolonged therapy is impressive and gives some credence to her explanations.

I believe that it may be possible to imagine that for some people the inability to let anything inside could also be seen as a fear of loss of the boundary of the self. Such a fear might range in severity from slight anxiety in those who can be helped in a few meetings, to an overwhelming panic in those whose vaginal spasm and protection of the interior of the body is a defence against psychotic breakdown.

I have recently had some clinical encounters that have supported the idea of a fear of loss of identity. One patient said, 'I have been alone for so long now that I cannot imagine what it would be like to be together with him.' She had in fact been married for 5 years. She identified her 'aloneness' as having started when she left home. Her marriage had in no way provided the sort of closeness that she had lost, or escaped from, when she left her parents' house.

The next patient had florid fantasies of the hymen right across the opening, with a long tunnel beyond in which things could get lost.

Case Study 21

Mrs Smith had suffered from severe eczema since babyhood. Her first memories were of having the bandages soaked off her legs by a visiting nurse. She had been seeing the psychosexual doctor every 2 or 3 weeks for about 6 months and was managing to examine herself vaginally with one finger, but complaining that she could not relax when she tried to make love. The doctor mused about her need to be in control and a possible fear of losing her sense of herself. She replied that this was the only area of her life that *was* under her control and that she felt that she had been persuaded into marriage. She had valued her freedom and felt safe by herself. The doctor remembered that her mother had had to cope by herself as her father had been away for the first 2 years of her life. Mrs Smith had felt that her father had been an intrusion when he came home.

During this meeting the patient was more thoughtful than she had been previously and did not need to be so briskly practical and sensible. During future meetings she was able gradually to take more control of herself and her efforts to come to terms with her body, and to encourage her husband to help her. She no longer wanted the doctor to examine her and was eventually happy to stop attending when the doctor moved away from the area. Three months later she achieved full intercourse with pleasure. Is it fanciful to suggest that she needed the doctor out of her vagina and her life before she could let her husband in?

The idea that every woman needs to 'own' her own vagina, take control of it from her mother before she can use it for intercourse, is well established. Her inability to do so may be mirrored in the relationship with her female doctor, who often becomes protective and instructive. Such a role is useful in order to explore and defuse frightening fantasies, but it does nothing to encourage independence. If it is not possible for the doctor to move to a relationship that can allow more separation, it may be necessary for the patient to change her therapist.[5] I believe we should not see such a move as a failure but as a finding that may help us to understand the underlying dynamics of her problem.

Some patients with vivid, hidden body fantasies show a strong need to be sensible, almost having a 'jolly hockeysticks' approach to their bodies. It is

easy to get captured by such a practical, no-nonsense atmosphere, in whic
any sign of weakness or silliness dare not show its face. A strong sense c
shame and self-hatred about her silly ideas may lead the patient to opt out c
treatment at an early stage. There is too a feeling that she must have 'goo
news' for the doctor, signs of progress, if she is to be entitled to further help

So far in this chapter I have been looking at some of the fears tha
women have about their own bodies. Although they are not conscious whe
the women start treatment, it is not too difficult to help them to voice thei
quite quickly. I do not think that these fantasies can be equated with thos
infantile misunderstandings that emerge during prolonged psychoanalysis, ye
verbalizing them within a therapeutic relationship that allows the patier
to progress from a protected, child-like role to one of independence, and
growing relationship with her partner, can allow consummation to take plac
in many cases. A prospective study of such work showed a consummation rat
of 60% in 6 months and 72% in 24 months.[6]

Eliciting the detail of a body fantasy may also be important when tryin
to help patients make sense of physical symptoms at different stages in the
lives.

Case Study 22

Mrs Short had visited her doctor several times since the birth of
her last child 2 years before, complaining of vaginal soreness and
painful intercourse. Candida had been cultured on some occasions but not others. At a recent meeting she said that until the last
few days she had been free of soreness for 6 months, but had not
wanted intercourse because she was always 'wet'.

The doctor knew she had some treatment at home that she
could use for the thrush and wondered to herself why she had
come. She suspected there were emotional problems and did a
slow, listening vaginal examination, during which the patient told
her that her husband said it was 'a disaster area'. She also said
that she herself felt it was 'like a funnel'. At that moment the doctor asked her to show her what she meant, and the patient sat up
and looked at her vulva, but became totally tongue-tied. 'I don't
know, I can't explain', she said, shaking her head and lying down
again.

When this case was discussed in a group it was interesting that half tl
members saw the funnel with the wide end downwards, perhaps suggesting a

over-stretched, baggy 'disaster area', while the other half saw it as having the narrow end down dripping the 'wetness' of which she complained. These two images could have very different meanings for the patient. The first might be associated with an idea of being overstretched by the baby, while the second could be concerned with something nasty inside producing the discharge. As the discussion continued, it became clear that the work of exploring her ideas about her body had been stopped by the act of looking at herself. Perhaps it is impossible to discover and formulate one's internal images of one's body when confronted by external ones.

I have often felt rather uncomfortable when doctors and other health care workers suggest that patients should look at themselves in a mirror, and now I think I understand why. The mental image needs to be brought into full consciousness and explored in detail before an attempt is made to confront reality. If patients themselves ask for a mirror, that may be the appropriate time to provide one.

A man too may have vivid fantasies about the vagina, which can express some of his feelings about the whole woman. The vagina may be disgusting or uninteresting, like rice pudding as one patient said,[7] or raw and easily damaged. There may be teeth inside, and if the partner is pregnant, the fantasy can be explained more easily as being the baby's teeth, even though the man realizes that the teeth could not really be formed and waiting to bite him within the vagina. The conflicting feeling that he could cause damage to the vagina and at the same time be damaged by it may be present in the same man, showing that he splits his feelings towards women, perhaps in the process keeping himself safe.

When thinking about sexual intercourse, the vagina is only one half of the equation. What about the penis that is to fill it? The woman who fears that her vagina is too small may see the erect penis as enormous. The power of such an excited and exciting organ can be felt as a threat, and a woman may say she is afraid it will take her over, or take him over, as if his passion is somehow contained in a penis that is unattached to him as a whole and loving person who could control it. Again the act of finding herself describing such feelings may make it easier for a woman to think about them with a more logical part of her mind. It may be helpful to discover whether it is the length or the girth of the penis which seems so big. More than one woman has said to me that she cannot imagine whether she could encircle it between her thumb and forefinger, and has gone home to try to see, thus taking her own decision to confront her fantasy with reality.

Having looked at some of the fantasies a woman can have about her body and that of her partner, and the man's feelings about the vagina, we come to the ideas the man may have about his own body, especially his penis. The fear that it is too small is of course well known, but it is worth wondering, too small for what? There may be a reciprocal fantasy of a large and insatiable woman/vagina.

The view that a man has of his own penis as he looks down on it may be obscured by a pad of suprapubic fat or by a protruding abdomen. This self view is different from that he gets of his father's, brother's or friend's equipment in the school shower. These are small matters compared with the sense of smallness as a man that can get fixed in the genital region. If the feelings about his bodily equipment can be discussed as part of his feeling about himself as a whole man, it may be possible for him to relocate his sense of smallness away from his penis and begin to deal with it in a more appropriate way.[8]

I wonder whether there may be almost as many fantasies about the foreskin as there are about the hymen.

Case Study 23

Mr Thomas was brought to a family planning clinic by his sexually experienced girlfriend. The complaint was that they could not make love and that he had a sore place on his penis. The doctor found an easily retractable foreskin and a small, clean abrasion at the base of the frenulum. Mr Thomas confessed that he had never been able to have intercourse, and referred vaguely to the fact that both the woman and the man had to be 'broken in'. It was not until the third visit that the doctor really listened to what he was saying and asked exactly what he meant. It became clear that he thought the foreskin had to be torn right back to the base of the penis. No wonder he kept getting a traumatic abrasion. Both patient and doctor were embarrassed by the misunderstanding, but now that he realized that the 'whole thing' was meant to go inside he managed easily.

It seems extraordinary that such misunderstandings still occur in a world with so much explicit and informal sex education and discussion, but he was a country lad who had learnt the facts of life from watching horses. Nevertheless, I think there must have been many other factors that contributed to his difficulties. Why, for example, did he imagine it had to be painful? In this case exploring the body fantasies alone was enough, but I believe there is much we do not know about what such ideas mean to the whole man.

Another patient who had never managed to make love remembers with great fear the first time his foreskin went back and he saw the glans. It seemed to him to be raw and revolting.

Such thoughts bring me back to the idea of mess and disgust, and the difficulty some people have in understanding how their body works in this emotionally charged region.

Case Study 24

Mr Uphill had never learnt the difference between the sensation of passing urine and ejaculating. He used to wet the bed as a child, and he had developed a technique of waking himself up if he had an erotic dream and then holding his penis until he reached the toilet. It was vital that he did not mark the sheets, be it with urine or semen. He had to collect the liquid in a jar and see whether it was cloudy before he could tell whether it was semen or not. The childhood cruelty that had led to such an inhibition was clear and almost overwhelming for the doctor, who could do little to help this otherwise most successful man. Would long-term psychotherapy have done so? Alas it was not available for him.

In this chapter I have looked at some of the fantasies, both conscious and unconscious, that people can have about their bodies that can interfere with love-making. Most of my examples have been taken from patients who have never been able to have intercourse, but for many others the confident use of their bodies can be undermined at other stages of their lives. Underlying some physical symptoms, for example of vaginal pain or dryness, testicular or penile pain, there may be mental images that lead the patient to locate some of their deep feelings about themselves on that part of the body. Throughout this book I have tried to think of a person as a total being, whose mind is influenced by the body's experiences and whose feelings may be translated into bodily sensations. Such a unified picture of the person is essential if we are to begin to understand the meaning of body fantasies and find ways of helping those whose sexual lives are crippled by them. Dr Tom Main taught that fantasies should be fully explored, valued, and then buried with full military honours.

References

1   Casement P (1985) *On Learning from the Patient*. Tavistock, London.

2   Main T (1989) The Institute and Psychoanalysis: Debt and differentiation. In *The Ailment and Other Psychoanalytic Essays* (ed. J Johns), Free Association Books, London.

3   McDougall J (1995) *The Many Faces of Eros*. Free Association Books, London.

4   McDougall J (1986) *Theatres of the Mind*. Free Association Books, London.

5   Skrine R (1994) Consummation and Non-consummation in the Doctor/ Patient Relationship. *Institute of Psychosexual Medicine Journal*. 7: 4.

6   Bramley M, Brown J, Draper K *et al.* (1983) Non-consummation of Marriage Treated by Members of the Institute of Psychosexual Medicine: a prospective study. *British Journal of Obstetrics and Gynaecology*. 90: 908.

7   Skrine R (1992) Sexuality and Body/Mind Doctoring. *Proceedings of the Institute of Psychosexual Medicine*. 1: 1–8.

8   Shepherd P (1994) 'I'm too Small.' *Institute of Psychosexual Medicine Journal*. 8: 14.

Sex, anger and the couple

It is the inner world of the partners and the nature of their interaction which determines their response to changing circumstances.

Diana Daniell[1]

I do not think I am alone in experiencing a sinking feeling when an individual or a couple says 'Everything is fine between us, it is just the sex.' In our Western culture towards the end of the twentieth century it is more acceptable to complain of sexual difficulties than of marital ones. If it is sexual, the problem may be physical, and it is then something that doctors should be able to treat.

There seems to be an extraordinary naivety about relationships and sex. Some young friends were recently talking to me about their plans and hopes, and they expressed the view that whatever else happened, they would make sure that the sex was all right before they committed themselves to a man. This is in many ways a sensible idea, because, as heterosexual women, they do not want to choose a man who, for example, is not very interested in women. But there appeared to be a belief that provided sex is all right at the beginning, it will remain that way for ever.

In a society where sexual experience early in relationships is the norm, one sees more and more people who cannot maintain their sexual interest once they begin to know their partner better. Some reasons for this were mentioned in Chapter 5, where I suggested that the shame of sexual feelings was easier to bear when the relationship was not very important, or where a man could remain in touch with his aggressive or 'dirty' sexuality when the girl did not matter.

Another common reason for a loss of sexual feeling and function is the inability to deal with negative emotions. It is difficult to get in touch with sexual feelings if one is feeling angry. What is anger about? Is it defensive, a need to protect one's inner vulnerability or sense of importance and self-worth? Why is it that couples find it so difficult to be straightforward with each other about what they feel and what they need emotionally?

There is now a great deal of experience and theoretical knowledge about how people react in relationships, and the unconscious reasons for partner choice and the use of each member by the other.[2] The Tavistock Institute of Marital Studies (TIMS) provides training and therapy which is of a high quality quite outside the scope of the ordinary body/mind doctor or the remit of this book. As doctors, some humility in our claims to understand the dynamics of relationships is in order, and I can do no more than touch on one or two issues in this chapter, referring the reader to more comprehensive texts.

Nevertheless, whether we like it or not, there will be many occasions on which we find ourselves faced by couples in trouble, and other times when we run away from the difficulty with one person by sending for the partner. The situation for the general practitioner can be complicated, as he often knows the partner in his or her own right. It can be difficult to separate that personal experience of the absent partner from the impression given by the patient in the room. If we do not know the partner, we can at least know that our feelings about the person we have never seen are coming to us from the present patient, and we can keep an open mind about how much is reality and how much is projection.

Each of us uses others to a greater or lesser degree to carry parts of ourselves that we are not able to own. Some relationships are collusive in the way that both partners project aspects of themselves into the other. For me, one of the most useful papers on mutual projection was written in 1986.[3] The husband of this couple appeared at first as weak, small and ineffectual, blaming his impotence on an earlier genital infection. In work with him it became clear that he projected aggressive aspects of himself into his wife and then hated them in her. She, on the other hand, had a great fear of her own weakness and ignorance, which she hated and projected into her husband in a castrating way. Work with them individually at first allowed each to contain more of the projected parts of themselves.

When faced with a couple I remember the adage I was given many years ago, that if there are two people in the room one can *only* concentrate on what is going on between them. Certainly, I have found it a safe and useful idea for such work, where the relationships between the couple and the doctor are so much more complicated than in the one-to-one situation. However, I am interested in Ruszczynski's observation that with some couples he is unable to think about or address them as a couple: 'I am more likely to get caught up with one of them'.[4] This spirit of observation and thoughtfulness about what *is* happening rather than generalized tips about what one *ought to be doing* is nearer the skill that interests me, but is a difficult one to acquire.

More pertinent to our work is the question of 'Who is the patient?' Often the complaining member of the couple convinces us that the one who is not there needs treatment. Yet experience shows us time and again that sending for the partner lands us with two patients, or one who does not wish to be there or to do any work. On the other hand, by staying with the patient who has come, one may be able to do something to help that patient contain more of those uncomfortable bits of him or herself that are being projected into the partner. The obvious difficulty is then one of blame. I often find myself saying very specifically that problems are always due to faults on both sides, but that relationships are complicated and that if one person can change even a little bit in a genuine way, that may help the partner to do so too, and natural momentum may do the rest. (Or not, alas, as is often the case.)

Case Study 25

Mr Osborne is the husband of Mrs Osborne described on p. 56. You may remember that she was unable to reach orgasm until she had remembered how her father called, 'You slut, you whore' from the bedroom window if she arrived home late when she was a teenager.

Mr Osborne had been the one to ask for help first. He had gone to his general practitioner and to his priest because he believed himself to be oversexed, wanting to make love every night, yet never feeling satisfied. Mrs Osborne, who had some insight into her own difficulties, was able to see that her problem might be contributing to his. After she learnt to reach orgasm, her husband found that he did not need to have sex so often, and they settled into a less frequent but much more satisfying pattern of love-making. It was as if her inability to enjoy herself fully had made him need to keep trying again and again, always being left unsatisfied but not knowing why. The psychosexual doctor never saw him herself, but learnt of the changes and the growth in his sense of self-worth and self-esteem from his wife.

This couple are interesting in that Mr Osborne at first located all the difficulty in himself, becoming so filled with guilt and shame that he felt the need of absolution from his priest. A more common situation is for the man to blame the woman for her lack of interest while denying that he could be playing any part in the situation or that their sex life could be related to their relationship.

I have to admit to a preference for working with single patients, for that is where the specific skills of a body/mind doctor seem to have most relevance and where I have most experience. Yet I have had to accept that if a couple want to come together, that says something about how they see their problem, and it is best to see them together. A review of my own practice in 1976 showed that I split up far more couples than I put together.[5] Now I try to resist that temptation, and offer what I can to them as they come. However, there are still some people who believe, as a lingering legacy of behavioural techniques, that couples must be seen together, and it is important to find out whether the referral has interfered with their own wishes.

A person who chooses to ask a doctor for help with what is reported as a marital problem may have hidden fears about the body and hidden difficulties with sexual arousal. It may be easier to talk about the nitty-gritty of sexual techniques with a doctor who is used to bodies, although that alone is unlikely to be of use unless the feelings are also explored.

Because of the complicated nature of the interaction between couples, I am looking in this chapter at just one important emotion, that of anger, and I shall give a few examples of how it interferes with sexual function.

Case Study 26

Mr Vine was brought to a family planning clinic by his girlfriend, and pushed into the room while she waited outside. He told the doctor how he used to be able to last for three quarters of an hour, but now he was so quick that sometimes he did not get inside at all before he ejaculated.

He told his story in a soft voice with a broad accent that made it difficult for the doctor to hear what he said. When asked to say a bit more about it he explained that they made love in his bedroom in his parents' home but denied that was a problem. His parents approved of his girlfriend and had liberal views. They all got on well, and his only complaint was about the family dogs.

There was a top dog and an under dog, and his mother always took the side of the top dog. It wasn't fair, but you couldn't say anything to women could you? The doctor asked, 'Why not?', and for the first time he looked at her directly and seemed thoughtful.

As he left the clinic with his girlfriend the doctor heard them beginning to argue, and at the next meeting he said things were back to normal.

Such an easy connection between unexpressed anger and sexual difficulty is seldom possible to make. The inhibitions against showing anger, or even feeling it, may lie deeply buried within the psyche. It is usually necessary for the patient to have some opportunity to experience anger within the therapeutic relationship, and have it tolerated, before he or she can begin to tolerate it internally. A fear of showing anger may be connected to memories of having lost control in such a way that someone was physically damaged or with the fear of causing serious damage. 'I could have killed him' is a common phrase. For such men there is much to be gained by seeing their sexual difficulty as being a physical problem with the body, and the differential diagnosis can be particularly difficult if there is some physical illness as well.

Case Study 27

Mr Walsh had been diagnosed as having multiple sclerosis, although at the time he sought help with his impotence his only physical complaint was that he could not run down escalators. He was getting good morning erections, but insisted that his impotence was due to his illness.

When invited to talk some more about the problem it became clear that he was furious with his wife, whom he portrayed as a bossy, complaining woman who had to be obeyed at all times. While paying lip service to the idea that he wanted to please her, he felt that nothing he did was ever right or good enough for her. Any suggestion that his impotence might be related to the relationship was strongly resisted, and the doctor was left feeling that nothing she could do or say would be good enough for this complaining, ingratiating man who kept thanking her for her time. He did not return for a second appointment.

There do not seem to be obvious reasons why one angry man develops premature ejaculation, another impotence and a third loss of sexual interest. All these symptoms can be frustrating for the partner, which may be what he unconsciously wants but which is strongly denied if interpreted directly. If he can be helped to express some of the anger, and any acting out in the therapeutic relationship can be tolerated, he may be able to make a change.

Containing the feelings without becoming retaliatory or conciliatory, or feeling destroyed, may not be easy for the doctor. Many of us have expressed our own unconscious drives by our very choice of career, which gives us an opportunity to push our neediness and uselessness into our patients. Our wish to make them better is very strong. The sense of impotence and uselessness can be hard to bear and may lead to inappropriate treatment with physical methods. The escape routes open to the doctor faced with an impotent man multiply with technical advances and now include vacuum devices, penile injections and prostheses. As the impotent despair of the patient becomes transferred to the doctor, the pressure to treat and 'make better' becomes acute (see the case of Mr Abbot on p. 6).

More doctors who are trained in psychosexual medicine are now offering penile injections as part of their own care of the patient. The physical treatment can then be understood as part of the ongoing therapeutic relationship, and becomes a matter for thoughtful study. It seems likely that patient satisfaction will be higher in these circumstances than where injections are offered merely as a hospital procedure akin to cystoscopy. It is interesting that in a urology-funded sexual problems clinic run by a general practitioner trained in psychosexual medicine, only 12.5% of men were given injections, although 89% of those who replied gave a positive response to a measure of satisfaction with the consultation.[6]

What of the angry woman? Again if the anger cannot be acknowledged she may remain sweet and compliant, believing herself happy in her relationship, yet inexplicably not wishing to have any sexual contact and not allowing any sexual feelings within herself. One of the most difficult things for her partner to believe is that this previously sexual woman now genuinely does not have or want such feelings. He believes that there must be something wrong with him or she must fancy someone else.

Case Study 28

Mrs Exe complained to her doctor that she had not wanted sex since the birth of her baby 2 years previously. Occasionally she did manage intercourse, for her husband's sake, and once she had an orgasm, but 'He had to drag it out of me', she said, and it gave her no pleasure.

In the consulting room Mrs Exe appeared defensively angry. She told the doctor how she had to fight for her 'rights' in several spheres of her life, particularly in relation to a family Will from which she had hoped for more money than she got. Yet behind the anger the tears were never far away. It was as if her attacking stance was all that stood between herself and some internal collapse.

When she talked about her husband she described a man who always had to be right. She had felt criticized by him for the way in which she handled the baby, and he seemed to need to win every argument. She could not see why she should make love if she did not want to, and she was adamant about that. The doctor suggested that sex was the one area in which she could still be in control, and that to 'give in' as she saw it would be to risk annihilation and loss of herself as an individual. This idea made sense to her and she began to see the problem as part of the marital relationship rather than just her body that was not working properly.

This case synopsis could have been used in Chapter 8 on sex and childbirth, as it was certainly the birth of the child that precipitated the problem. Yet the angry fear of being taken over by her husband's forcefulness, a characteristic that may have been what attracted her to him in the first place (in the hope that he could control her own aggression?) was not necessarily dependent on the baby. It could have arisen at any time as the relationship progressed beyond the 'first fine careless rapture' to something deeper, where negative feelings had to be tolerated.

Such anger may present to a doctor as physical pain, particularly vaginal pain on intercourse. You may remember Mrs Farrell on p. 20 who said early in the consultation, 'I know and you know why I have the pain.' In fact the doctor had no idea, but the patient went on to say immediately that she was cross and did not want to make love. Strangely, she only needed to hear herself saying that to the doctor to be able to go home and begin to sort out the relationship. Another woman, who tended to accept a scapegoat role in her relationship with a rather silent, self-absorbed man, told of how she had been lying in bed quite unable to get in touch with any sexual feelings. Suddenly she found herself saying angrily to herself, 'Tomorrow I will *make* him listen to me', and immediately her body began to respond.

The cause of the anger is always specific for the individual and reverberates with earlier experiences. Sometimes the patient makes connections with the past quite easily if allowed to go back and remember in her or his own way, rather than trying to search the memory in order to answer a doctor's questions.

Case Study 29

Mr Young was complaining of lack of sexual interest associated with some difficulty with erection. He was protective of his new, second wife, who was in the waiting room during the discussion, and he made the doctor feel that she had to be careful not to imply that the wife could be in any way to blame.

After an easy and normal physical examination Mr Young admitted to getting nocturnal and morning erections, but said he was ashamed of them: 'They don't seem like proper erections, I ought to be able to control them.' He went on to tell the doctor how, during a school medical examination when he was 12, he had developed a partial erection and the doctor had said he should 'control himself'. Despite this he had always been able to respond to attractive women, but now his new wife did not approve of him looking at other women. It was difficult for him to value his sexuality, and for them both to accept that there could be sexual arousal in response to phantasy that he did not wish to act upon and that did not pose a threat to their relationship. The doctor felt that the passive acceptance of the wife's strictures, and the inability to fight for what was normal and natural within himself, was more likely to threaten the marriage.

In the consultation the clues to the important ideas and memories will be the emotional force in the patient and the feelings in the doctor. Snatching at explanations that do not have emotional force may be reassuring but suggests that they are being used as a defence against more painful feelings. As Lincoln puts it, 'The defence of love and happiness protects the psyche from the pain of recognising the bad feelings and the despair which might put the relationship in serious jeopardy.' And later in the same chapter 'the need is for the doctor to follow the patient beyond what may appear to be an adequate explanation ... to whatever point of deep emotional pain the patient may discover.'[7]

Several central concepts about marriage have emerged from the work of TIMS, and I can do no more than just mention them here. The relationship is seen as being a psychic entity in itself, a system greater than the sum of the personalities of the partners.[7] The choice of partner reflects unconscious needs, and when things begin to go wrong it is often the unwanted and projected bits of themselves that they hate in the other.[8] Such a change often occurs when one partner changes or matures at a different rate from the other. The collusive interaction that has worked reasonably well begins to break down, and problems in their sexual life may well be a presenting symptom. It is here that the doctor may be approached with a number of unspoken or even unconscious aims.

The most rewarding patients are those who have genuinely not made a connection between their sexual problem and the relationship. Within an open consultation that may have started with a physical symptom or sexual complaint, a torrent of anger against the partner may suddenly surprise the patient as much as the doctor. For example, one woman whose mother's death was soon followed by the death of her dog became furious with her husband who did not seem to understand her 'irrational' wish for another dog.[7] It seemed here that it was the anger with him for not understanding her feelings rather than the bereavement itself that was inhibiting her sexual response. (I notice that two cases that I have chosen to use in this chapter have included dogs! Is this another version of the 'kick the cat' syndrome – displaced feelings that can be tolerated more easily within oneself if directed towards animals rather than people?)

A doctor may quite often be asked for help with a sexual problem not because genuine change is wanted, but to show the partner that everything that could be done has been. 'I went to the doctor but he couldn't help me' locates the problem firmly outside him or herself and may make the acceptance of the breakdown easier. There may already have been a decision to end the relationship taken by one person but not yet shared with the partner. Identifying such a situation may save the doctor a lot of time. Yet even here the motivation may not be as straightforward as it seems. Underneath there may be hidden anxieties and self-blame about the breakdown, and worries about the chances of making a satisfactory relationship in the future. If the doctor can take a neutral moral stance, it is surprising how often underlying worries about sexual adequacies, even bodily failings such as a small penis or lack of sexual attractiveness, will surface at this time of crisis.

Theories of marital function and dysfunction such as those mentioned briefly above can be rather daunting for the ordinary doctor, but I believe we can have a useful part to play if we stay with the person in the room and with the body/mind work with which we are familiar. One of our handicaps is our need to be active and 'therapeutic'. In the face of a patient who has difficulties expressing or containing anger, there is a temptation to retaliate, retreat or become very active. Angry feelings within ourselves need to become the subject of study, not as some sort of personal therapy, but as a useful tool in understanding our patients.

Writing this chapter has given me some difficulty. Although I and my colleagues see many patients whose inability to deal with their anger inhibits their sexual lives, they have not sprung readily to mind. How much easier it is as a doctor to write about loss, vulnerability and shame, than to celebrate anger, excitement and joy. Yet these are necessary parts of a full emotional life. When working in psychosexual training seminars I value the occasional member who can identify and tolerate negative feelings, for they can free us from our hidden aggression. Alas there are not many doctors blessed with this gift, and of course those who allow their anger to spill out in a destructive way are no more help. I have to recognize my own difficulty with anger as a personal trait that can inhibit my doctoring as well as my writing. I do so here because I believe that many in the helping professions share such traits, and they can lead to what Main[9] has called velvet doctoring:

> *Let us say ... that the doctor is concerned to be seen as kind, sweet, loving, sympathetic, sensitive, tactful, wise and unabrasive; the kind of doctor to which we all aspire to be – and which none of us is! The worst instances concern those doctors who are so afraid of being aggressive that they have velvet thoughts, velvet voices, velvet techniques and often velvet interpretations. Their clinical techniques are seriously limited by their fear of being aggressive.*

We hope that the experience of work in a structured group will allow doctors to see not their personal hang-ups about their aggressiveness, but the way in which these may be interfering with their ability to help patients. If we can identify some of the hidden hostility that patients bring to the consultation, contain it, think about and understand it, they may be better able to cope with such feelings in their personal relationships.

References

1   Daniell D (1985) The Psychodynamic Approach. In *Marital Therapy in Britain* (ed. W Dryden), Harper & Row, London.

2   Salzberger-Wittenberg I (1970) *Psychoanalytic Insights and Relationships.* Routledge, London.

3   Main T (1986) Mutual Projection in Marriage. *Comprehensive Psychiatry.* 5: 432–49.

4   Ruszczynski S (1995) Narcissistic Object Relating. In *Intrusiveness and Intimacy in the Couple* (eds. S Ruszczynski and J Fisher), Karnac, London.

5   Skrine R (1976) Who Is the Patient? In *Practice of Psychosexual Medicine* (ed. K Draper), J Libbey, London.

6   Stainer-Smith A (1996) Dare we Measure Patient Satisfaction? *Institute of Psychosexual Medicine Journal.* 12: 11–14.

7   Lincoln R (1992) Loss of Libido. In *Psychosexual Medicine* (ed. R Lincoln), Chapman & Hall, London.

8   Clulow C (1985) *Marital Therapy: An inside view*. Aberdeen University Press, Aberdeen.

9   Main T (1987) In *Psychosexual Training and the Doctor/Patient Relationship* (ed. R Skrine), p. 33. Chapman & Hall, London.

Sex and childbirth

Psychic reality dictates the meaning of childbirth rather than external reality.
Raphael-Leff[1]

The birth of every child is a momentous occasion in the life of individuals and families. It is a moment of great potential for emotional growth, when there is the possibility for readjustments within the individual and between couples. At the same time the heightened emotional climate that provides the opportunity for such growth opens the door to pain and vulnerability that can have profound and long-lasting effects, particularly in the sexual areas of people's lives.

All the emotions that have been mentioned so far in this book, such as shame, anger and grief, can be aroused by the experiences of pregnancy, childbirth and the process of becoming a parent. Perhaps underlying all of them is the knowledge that where there is a potential for new life, there is always the possibility that things can go wrong. There can be sudden death or the birth of a less than perfect child. If one opens one's heart to love, there is always the possibility of loss.

It is, of course, artificial to separate out, as I have done in this book, emotions that are almost always found together. I hope that this contrived simplicity will not lead the doctor to jump to rapid conclusions based on preconceived ideas, but will go some way in helping us to untangle the detail of feeling for each person. The skill must always be to wait in ignorance with the patient until some real feeling emerges. Such an approach is particularly true when we consider emotions relating to childbirth, as the experience resonates with the very deepest levels of the personality of each one of us. The growing fetus within, followed by the arrival of the helpless, newborn infant, sets off reverberations in the unconscious which may be concerned with the mother herself as a very young child, or with her memories of the birth of a sibling, or other early painful experiences.[2]

A word of caution. Some patients date the change in their sexual life to the birth of a child. Further discussion may reveal that there were many other changes taking place at the same time. Some couples may only start to live together or to get married when pregnancy occurs. Often the woman gives up her job and has to face loneliness and isolation as well as all the other changes associated with a new, close and, as it were, full-time relationship. Many people remain in touch with their sexual feelings while the relationship is new and spiced with frequent partings and meetings, as was discussed in the previous chapter. Such feelings will be mixed with the deeper and older psychological factors. Untangling the many different changes and the effect on each individual person is a complicated piece of detection, needing close observation of the details of the moment by moment happenings in the consulting room.

In Table 8.1 I have listed some of the subject areas that come up during discussions with a psychosexual doctor following childbirth, but as with all the tables in this book I must emphasize once again that there is no attempt to be comprehensive. All such lists can do is to suggest one or two signposts that patients may be trying to use, often without realizing it, to point towards their difficulty as they struggle to understand baffling changes in their feelings. The table was prepared with the woman in mind, and I present it here in that way, but as I look at it I realize that I have seen men too who share many of these anxieties.

Any health care worker who has licence to examine the genital area must be aware of the possible physical problems associated with perineal tears, episiotomies and genital infections. Sometimes it is not easy to say categorically that it is physically normal, and indeed the interplay of mind and body is

Table 8.1:   Some factors in postpartum sexual problems

Sore perineum
Fantasies
  e.g. of damage
  Too small
  Too big
Unresolved feelings about the delivery
  Failure as a woman
  Memory of exposure or sense of attack
  Associating vagina with pain rather than pleasure
Interest and emotion centred on the baby – husband shut out
Jealousy of the baby
Difficulty reconciling role as mother and lover
Postnatal depression

nowhere more crucial. The tender scar that causes pain on the first attempted intercourse and is then pulled forward by protective muscle spasm on all further attempts so that it is, as it were, offered for further trauma, is very common. Detailed examination of the introitus may show that the pain is anterior, with tenderness behind the pubic bone. Simple explanations about the importance of contracting the pelvic floor before trying to relax it may be enough if given as part of a listening, empathetic examination.

The interaction at such an intimate moment is often concerned with giving back the control of her own body to the woman. She may have felt at some specific moment during the delivery that she lost control. If this loss is associated with a feeling of vulnerability or violation, the experience can remain in the mind, haunting her for many months or years. The fact that the violation was usually some clinically necessary procedure, done with the best intentions in her interest and that of her baby, does not help if the woman's past experiences have sensitized her to such happenings.

Case Study 30

Mrs Z had been unable to enjoy her sexual life since the birth of her baby 4 years previously. When talking about her preparation for the birth she described how important it had been for her to go to the antenatal classes with her husband and how much they had both been looking forward to the birth experience. All went well at first. Then she had an internal examination that was very painful and she felt as if she had been attacked. She says she heard the midwife say afterwards that she had a low pain threshold, and this added to her sense of helplessness and fury.

Over the course of three meetings it became clear that Mrs Z had come into the pregnancy potentially vulnerable. Her father had left home when she was 6, her mother had suffered from a manic–depressive illness and much of the responsibility for her younger brother had been carried by Mrs Z since she was 12 years old. In particular she had learnt not to trust her mother, as promised treats never materialized. Only by remaining in control of her own feelings and not allowing herself to hope could she protect herself from disappointment.

She had done well after she left school, training for a managerial job at which she excelled. The sense of competence in her work gave her much pleasure, and she had looked forward to embracing motherhood in the same way. Her sudden sense of vulnerability to a powerful and, as she experienced it, uncaring older woman opened up many old wounds. At the time of the examination her husband had been sent out of the room, but her anger that he had not protected her from the 'attack' was in no way helped by her intellectual understanding that he had to do as he was asked. Now her fear of the vulnerability of sexual arousal was combined with her sense that her husband had betrayed her, and there was no way she could allow him to get close.

With the doctor too she needed to be in control, both of the timing of the physical examination and of every detailed step they took together. She appeared to get some relief from the interpretation of her fear of losing control, but remained in charge by deciding not to return for a fourth meeting with the doctor.

For Mrs Z there was a specific vulnerability to desertion by a man: she had, after all, been deserted by her father at the age of 6, which she was unlucky enough to have replayed during the delivery. Her husband's absence during what felt like an abusive intrusion by an untrustworthy woman must have reawakened her old feelings of panic when she was left to cope with her manic–depressive mother without the help of her father. No wonder she needed to keep control.

Sometimes the damage may be felt in a more physical way and become fixed as a body fantasy. Such fantasies can sometimes be seen to represent the emotional change that has occurred within herself as a result of becoming a mother. The vagina that feels like a 'wellington boot' could be an image of someone who is now so huge in her role as a mother that she cannot also be the firm, exciting and excited lover of previous times.

The very words we use may play into a fantasy and become a nidus for a misunderstanding, for example the phrase 'sewn up'.

Case Study 31

Mrs Atkins had not made love for 3 years since the birth of her first baby, and had already had one perineal repair and was on the waiting list for a second one. The psychosexual doctor managed to insert three fingers easily and so did the patient. Following this self-examination, she managed intercourse, and at the second meeting the doctor was about to congratulate her and show her to the door. Something in the patient's manner made her hesitate, and after a pause Mrs Atkins said, 'I suppose if it had been stitched up as I imagined, after six babies there would be no hole left.' As she was saying this her hand was making a movement as if she was cobbling up a hole in a stocking.

If the body fantasy had not been explored, it is possible that her mental images would have overridden the experience of her exploring fingers, and of the penis inside, and the sense of being too small might have resurfaced. We have evidence of the strength of her fantasy in the fact that she was on the waiting list for a further operation. We need to understand the power such fantasies can have on us, rather than just blaming colleagues for their blindness.

Husbands are just as vulnerable to the birth experience and may be left with their own private fantasies about the changes that have taken place in their wives' bodies. Watching the birth process produces complicated emotions that may need to be explored in detail. The memories are often crystal clear, even after many years. One man was given his baby to hold, but felt he missed out on an important bonding moment because he could think of nothing apart from the obstetrician's hands inside his wife as he stitched her up. Another was full of guilt about the damage that he felt had been done to his wife's body, and he took all the blame onto himself as the cause of the pregnancy. Both these men had trouble becoming actively sexual after the birth, and for both the upset seemed much greater than for their wives.

It is still difficult to take adequate care of the husband or partner in the labour ward and afterwards. Perhaps it is the English temperament that makes it so difficult for a man to admit that he would prefer not to be present or to leave the room if he wants to do so. Some say they must stay for their wife's sake, and feel that if she can cope with the experience, he should be able to be at least as brave. The very real emotional strain that some men subject themselves to for the sake of their wives, or in order not to lose their self-esteem, cannot be overestimated. That is not to deny that for many men the experience of childbirth can be a deeply satisfying and rewarding one. We need to develop a culture in which it is as legitimate for a man to choose how much or how little he wants to be present at the birth as it is for the woman to choose the type of labour she wants.

If such individual freedoms are to be arranged, there must be an atmosphere of flexibility between the couple, and women must be helped to understand the importance and possible damage that watching the birth can have on a man and therefore on their future relationship.

Sometimes there can be a joint fantasy, where it is impossible to tell from which person the idea first started. Perhaps it does not matter if they come together and the image is treated as one that belongs to them both.

Case Study 32

Mr and Mrs Ball came asking for an operation to remove the awful episiotomy scar that was making sex impossible. The doctor asked them to tell her a bit about the problem, and there followed a long and anguished account of a disappointing delivery. It seemed that everything had been going well until the second stage. They had planned the conception to coincide with their financial stability, had attended antenatal classes and arranged to have the doctor and midwife they trusted. However, in the second stage the doctor was called away to an emergency and Mrs Ball was delivered by a stranger. That was not all. As her episiotomy was being repaired a more senior doctor came past and said it was not being done properly and must be undone and resewn.

They went on to describe the horrendous scar, and the doctor prepared herself to see something shocking. When she looked she could not believe the thin, white, hardly visible scar, with a tiny dimple at one end. There was no way that further surgery could possibly have made any improvement, and indeed it might well have made the final result worse.

For this rather perfect couple the trauma of the delivery had become fixed in both their minds on the perineum. It is perhaps hard to sympathize with the extent of their distress, as by many standards the trauma was not great and they had got a perfect baby. Yet it seems that the sudden loss of control by two people who managed their life together by controlling it had been a serious upset. Perhaps being such 'sensible' people the only way in which they could deal with their combined sense of damage was by feeling it on her body.

Shame and guilt may be present in relation to the birth experience, especially if either member of the couple feels they did not perform very well. In favourable circumstances the vulnerability of the actual birth is quickly forgotten in the excitement of receiving the baby. Women will say that even by the next day they are beginning to regain their sense of privacy, for example when it comes to intimate examinations. If the birth experience is traumatic, the situation can be very different. It is important to try to separate out the feeling of shame, as if it is not dealt with by some form of 'debriefing' it can be felt for many years afterwards.

Case Study 33

Miss Clark went to her doctor complaining of painful intercourse ever since the birth of her only child 8 years before. She described what was for her a grim experience of a forceps delivery, saying frequently that if only she had been a better woman it would have been all right. The sense of not being a good enough woman had got fixed in her pelvis, and now she was demanding a hysterectomy to take the bad bits of herself away. When the doctor finally suggested that perhaps the baby had been lying the wrong way round and could not have been born naturally, the patient looked up for the first time. 'You mean it may not have been all my fault?', she said.

Alas for this patient it was too late to change her belief and she went ahead with the hysterectomy. On this occasion the shame was not to do with a fear of being too sexual, as has been discussed in Chapter 5, at least not overtly, but rather of being hopeless as a woman. However, the anxiety about humiliation, the exposure of being no good and the fear of rejection were all clear in the consultation.

Midwives, health visitors and doctors are now much more aware of the need for some sort of review of a labour when it is over, but there is still some misunderstanding of what is meant by 'debriefing'. Dictionary definitions include 'to gather information from a soldier, astronaut etc. on his return from a mission; to relive an experience with someone else to make sense of it'. The patient may want to know what actually happened, but a far more important job is to try and find out what it felt like to her, as the quotation at the head of this chapter suggests.

Further debriefing at a later date is often needed. In my work I do not usually see women till at least 6 weeks after delivery, when they have had time to organize their ideas about the experience. Do some women need time to integrate their memories and weigh them against their previous experience before they can really make sense of them? I certainly see many women, and some men too, who have carried the scars that have grown inside for many years, as the case of Miss Clark illustrates. For many people the scar is hidden from their awareness and may only show itself in a sexual dysfunction. By the time that help is sought the relationship may have deteriorated beyond repair.

The importance of discovering with the patient what the delivery meant to her is highlighted by the idea proposed by Raphael-Leff that women approach pregnancy in two different ways, as facilitators or regulators.[1] She stresses that there are few 'pure types' but that women gravitate towards one or other pole of the continuum. The facilitator gives in to the emotional upheaval of pregnancy, while the regulator tries to control it. Despite the suggestion from the names used that the facilitator might be somehow 'better' than the regulator the author points out that both can get into emotional trouble, but the feelings within the woman will be different and will be springing from different roots.

The sense of failure with regard to the delivery and postnatal period is felt differently by the two types of woman. The facilitator mother feels a failure when her idealized unrealistic standards of mothering cannot be achieved. For the regulator her self-esteem and sense of adult competence can be eroded by the baby who fails to become 'regulated'.[1] Perhaps such women are particularly at risk when they feel out of control or attacked. Mrs Z, the first woman described in this chapter (on p. 92), can be seen as someone who had to regulate all aspects of her life in order to remain safe and whose loss of control during delivery remained etched on her memory. Miss Clark, on the other hand, appears to have been particularly badly affected by a forceps delivery that left her feeling it was all her fault for not being a better woman, and the guilt and sense of failure gave her physical pain that culminated in a hysterectomy 8 years later.

Neither of these women remembered having talked about their experiences in any detail, and it is tempting to blame the system for not providing such an opportunity. It may be that they were offered help but the task of getting in contact with or reliving the feelings was too great or the patient's defences at the time were too strong. Such a failure highlights the need for all health professionals and counsellors to have their ears continually open so that small moves towards a search for help at a later date can be picked up. For both these women their plea for help eventually surfaced years later as a sexual problem.

The presenting symptom of complicated intra- and interpersonal changes may be a male sexual problem. Raphael-Leff suggests a continuum in men, parallel to that in women, from the renouncer, who distances himself from as many of the processes of childbirth as possible, to the participator, who may even feel jealous of the mother's immediate relationship with the baby.[1] The outcome will depend on how well the characteristics of the two parents dovetail together.

Case Study 34

Mr and Mrs Davies came to a psychosexual clinic because they wanted a second child and he had not been able to ejaculate in the vagina since the birth of their daughter 3 years previously. That birth and perinatal period had been fraught with problems. The baby was induced at 37 weeks because of maternal hypertension and was in intensive care for the first 4 weeks. Mrs Davies sat by the baby for most of that time as she felt that the baby knew when she was not there and would blame her for desertion when she grew up. Mr Davies felt isolated and shut out, although his wife blamed him for not being more help: 'I was left to do it all', she said.

In discussion with the doctor Mr Davies took an active part, and it was striking how differently each of them remembered the experiences. For Mrs Davies it was the immediate postnatal period that was most difficult, but Mr Davies had found the pregnancy hard. He felt that his wife turned to her mother for support rather than to him. Her mother had always been particularly protective following a serious illness that Mrs Davies had in childhood. 'It is difficult for me to get in', he said.

The situation between them was made worse by her conviction that he had lost interest in her sexually because she had gained weight. Somehow, however hard she tried, she could not feel good enough. In fact his sexual interest was as great as ever, with good erections and sexual feelings, but he was not able to finish the act.

When listening to this story I was reminded of the study of men who were unable to ejaculate in the vagina and the suggestion that there could be unconscious rivalry with the potential child.[3] It appeared that Mr Davies came from a rather 'distant' family, and the experience of being shut out by the mother, daughter and baby triad reverberated with earlier feelings of exclusion. The possibility of yet another baby must have reawakened those painful feelings, and although consciously wanting another child, his body was responding by making it impossible.

Perhaps one could see Mr Davies as someone whose past experience conditioned him to be a renouncer yet who desperately wanted to be a participator. Mrs Davies seemed to be a facilitator who had to face overwhelming practical difficulties with her baby that aroused deep feelings of guilt and inadequacy. The strong feelings on both sides made it difficult to re-establish a close relationship.

Memories of losing control during the birth process, with all the anxiety or fear that such a feeling can produce, may affect the sexual life of a man as seriously as that of a woman. Some men have been sensitized to the need to maintain control by earlier experiences. Sexual activity demands some loss of control if it is to work satisfactorily, and postnatal impotence may occur if the birth experience was traumatic for the man. Sometimes the sense of helplessness in the face of overwhelming anxiety about his wife, the baby or both, tunes in to earlier memories when he had to take responsibility beyond his capacities.

Case Study 35

Mr Edwards talked of the sudden death of his father when he was 8 years old. He had two younger brothers, and in the face of his mother's collapse when his father died he felt he had to take control of the family. One night he was found wandering about the house planning how he would have to sell it if they were to have enough money to live. With the help of grandparents and friends the family appeared to make a reasonable recovery, and when Mr Edwards grew up he got a good job in a bank.

At the time of his wife's first pregnancy there was some uncertainty about the future of his job. Added to the financial worry the birth was a particularly unhappy experience for him. His memory is of being left alone with his wife for long periods, not knowing how to help her. During a prolonged second stage he became convinced that his wife and/or the baby were going to die. His subsequent impotence could be seen as a way of protecting himself from the pain and anxiety of a similar experience.

In the first few weeks following delivery the mother meets the demands of her baby to the best of her ability. Some mothers can give themselves over to 'primary maternal preoccupation',[4] where the interest in the new baby excludes everything else. Such a woman may feel any sexual interest that her partner shows as an intrusion into an almost magical bond. The less fortunate mother may experience what has been called 'primary maternal persecution',[5] and for her a sexual approach is just one more demand that saps her strength and her sense of self.

As the weeks go by the intensity of those early reactions is modified, but the mother's awareness of her baby may still make it impossible for her to 'let go' in sexual abandonment, as this can feel as if she is abandoning the baby. The fear is that she might not hear the baby, or be there for it, if she allowed herself the momentary loss of awareness of herself, for some women a feeling akin to loss of consciousness, that is associated with orgasm.

One or both of the parents may have complicated feelings about her body, especially her breasts and vagina, as being for the baby rather than for them to use for sexual pleasure. The physical sequelae of the pregnancy and birth must be assessed and taken seriously by the body/mind doctor. Factors such as vaginal dryness in the breast-feeding mother are real and important. At the same time the feelings about the changes will colour their perception. Many women blame their lack of sexual responsiveness on increased weight, stretch marks or general lack of attractiveness. Reassurance from their partner does little to allay their disgust with their own body. They will say, 'How can he find me attractive?' It can feel to the woman as if his ability to find her sexy in the face of her own discontent with her body makes him into some kind of 'dirty old man', someone who would like any woman, just wanting physical relief for himself, rather than as an expression of love for her as an individual.

We come finally to the problem of postnatal depression and its inter-action with sexual feelings. The subject is complicated, not least because there are different views about the aetiology of postnatal depression, with horm-onal and psychoanalytic explanations both having a part to play. It seems likely that the illness is due to the interaction of several different factors. This book is not the place for a detailed discussion of these issues, but it is clear that the early diagnosis and appropriate treatment of postnatal depression is extremely important. Too many cases are still missed and women are left to struggle on in isolation.

Loss of sexual interest is cited as one of the signs of depressive illness, but the sense of losing one's sexual feelings can in itself generate feelings of depression and lack of self-worth. The sexual problem may persist long after the depression itself has been treated satisfactorily. Despite the classical descrip-tion some women continue to be able to respond sexually when depressed, and I have met one or two whose sexual problem only started as they began to recover from the depression. Perhaps for them there was something about the dependency of their illness which allowed them to hand control to their partner and let go sexually. Clearly, the processes at work are complicated and not fully understood.

For the professional who is trying to help it is important to take the sexual problem seriously. It may be necessary to treat the depression first, as brief interpretive work is usually not appropriate when the patient is seriously depressed. However, it should not be dismissed, and opportunities for discussion about the sexual problem should be arranged when the patient feels she wishes to discuss it, not postponed indefinitely with the reassurance that it will 'get better in time'. Unfortunately, such spontaneous improvement does not always happen, and the patient should at least have the chance to try to understand herself further if that is what she wants to do.

The next chapter looks further at some of the effects of grief on sexual life, but here I will just mention the question of hidden grief that may be present even at the time of successful and happy childbirth. There are, of course, the obvious difficulties associated with the loss of a loved one during the perinatal period, or the loss of one twin during a pregnancy and the survival of the other. As Tobert has said, 'To feel the sadness of death and the gladness of birth imposes a severe emotional challenge'.[2] For some women there is the knowledge that this has to be the last baby, perhaps for health or economic reasons, and the sense that they have lost their future reproductive life at the moment when it is most intensely present can be hard indeed. The feeling of being within a body that is so obviously ageing and being changed can remind some women of their own mortality. Thus the feelings that can be aroused by childbirth may echo back to their own earliest days as a dependent infant or provoke thoughts of the future, including their own demise.

References

1   Raphael-Leff J (1991) *Psychological Processes of Childbearing*. Chapman & Hall, London.

2   Tobert A (1992) Pregnancy Childbirth and Female Sexuality. In *Psychosexual Medicine* (ed. R Lincoln), Chapman & Hall, London.

3   Lincoln R and Thexton R (1983) Retarded Ejaculation. In *Practice of Psychosexual Medicine* (ed. K Draper), J Libbey, London.

4   Winnicott D W (1956) *Through Paediatrics to Psychoanalysis*. Hogarth Press, London.

5   Raphael-Leff J (1986) Facilitators and Regulators: Conscious and unconscious processes in pregnancy and early motherhood. *British Journal of Medical Psychology*. 59: 43.

9

Loss and vulnerability

The reaction of grief in response to loss is an intensely personal one, and each one of us has to negotiate mourning of our losses in his or her own way. There is only so much pain that the individual can bear, and psychological defence systems come into play to try to protect the person from being overwhelmed. If these measures fail, there is a risk of physical breakdown or even death. Loss of a partner is known to be one of the most severe forms of psychological stress.[1]

In this chapter I am considering not only the loss of loved ones, when there is a recognition and expectation of grief, but in addition those less obvious losses that are part of the experience of human living, but which may not be recognized as losses by the patient or valued by the doctor. Unless they are recognized they cannot be mourned and laid aside.

Abandonment to sexual pleasure happens in a different way for each person and may be a different experience on one occasion from that on another. The sense of such abandonment often feels like an opening to vulnerability and to the possibility of being hurt or ridiculed, as has been shown in some of the cases quoted in this book. The protective defences that come into play against unbearable grief may, despite conscious wishes to the contrary, interfere with sexual responsiveness. Coombs has said, 'The experience of mourning has to do with the constant remembering of the lost one. Arousal and orgasm have something to do with the forgetting of the outside world, and are often not permitted by those who mourn'.[2] I must emphasize that the prohibition is an internal one.

To abandon one's body and emotions to another requires great trust and involves an opening to feelings and the risk of breaking through protective barriers. However, the vulnerability is two-fold. The opening of oneself to the painful feelings within, the sense of loss that has been sealed away so that it can be prevented from destroying the personality, may be even more of a threat than opening up to a sexual partner.

For some the breaking of barriers can be a relief and comfort. Partners whose sexual life has been a mutual delight and succour may find that sex is a particularly potent way of providing and receiving comfort in times of sorrow. The relief of sexual tension may produce a flood of tears and anguish that could not be released in other ways, thus providing an opportunity for the partner to share the pain, and comfort and hold his or her bereaved partner. For such solace to be possible both individuals need to be able to tolerate their sense of vulnerability and helplessness to some extent.

For many people the defences against such inner neediness are very strong, and the fight to survive cuts them off from many of their deeper emotions. I am surprised how often the link between some personal loss and a sexual problem has not been considered, and it is often not until a patient talks about the other things that were going on in his or her life at the time the problem started that the connection is made. The dissociation creates an important technical point in psychosexual work. If patients are asked what they think might have caused the problem, there is usually a blank response. They have after all been asking themselves that question and would not have come to a doctor if they could have discovered the answer. Such a question deserves the answer 'That is what I have come to you to find out.' If the same problem is approached by wondering out loud what else was going on in the patient's life at that time, then a conscious connection is not demanded and the mind is freed to roam more widely.

It is not uncommon for the grief and associated sexual difficulty to present as a bodily problem. The following case was first reported in the *Journal of Sexual and Marital Therapy*.

Case Study 36

Mrs Ford went to a family planning clinic asking for a cervical smear. She told the doctor that she was already on the waiting list to see a gynaecologist because she was getting pain on intercourse. When the doctor asked about the pain she said, 'Well, we don't do it much now.' The doctor enquired when the pain had started, and she said, 'About 6 months ago.' 'What else was going on at that time?', the doctor asked. Mrs Ford burst into tears and said her father had died. The doctor provided tissues and they talked about how close she had been to her father and how she missed him. After about 10 minutes the doctor took the smear and found a retroverted uterus, which was slightly tender to the touch. She explained this finding to the patient, who confirmed that the pain was the same as that she felt during intercourse.

While the doctor did the paperwork the patient dressed behind the screen in the same room. Suddenly she called out, 'I think I have always had that pain, but I used to be able to wriggle around and make it all right. Now that I hurt all over it is just the last straw.'

For this patient it was important that the person who examined her body was also interested in her feelings, as she was then able to put the two together. She took her name off the surgical waiting list, and in due time, when she had recovered from the acute grief of her father's death, she was able to enjoy love-making again without pain.

Men too can feel their emotional pains in their bodies, and it is possible that we are missing many of these cases. In society today men are still not encouraged to show their feelings to any great extent, and unless doctors can develop the skill of helping them to make links between the body and the mind, they will continue to suffer bodily ills and perhaps be subjected to physical treatments that are not needed or appropriate.

Case Study 37

Mr Goddard complained of testicular pain and attended a genito-urinary clinic, where the examination and all tests were found to be normal. The doctor wondered what his present situation was, and she was told that his fiancée, who was still in his home country on the other side of the world, was pressing him to get married. He had come to England to work for a limited time, but although he loved her very much, he had decided to extend his stay away from home. The doctor looked enquiring, and he burst out that he could not bear to go home at the moment as he was still missing his grand-mother so much. She had recently died, and as he talked about how she had been the most important woman in his life, he surprised himself by starting to cry. At his next visit he talked again about his grandmother, but there was no further mention of testicular pain.

For this man the emotional pain had expressed itself through his body. It was almost as if his testis was being squeezed between the two women that he loved, and he could not commit himself to his girlfriend until he had properly mourned his grandmother.

The problem of impotence in a new relationship after the death of a wife is so common as to be known colloquially as 'widower's droop'. Again there may have been inadequate grieving. Many men, especially in their later years, seem to rush into new relationships. Perhaps there is a sense that time is passing them by and of wanting to find happiness before it is too late. The feelings for each man will be different and will contain a whole mixture of emotions. A sense of betrayal and unfaithfulness to the dead partner may be strongly denied yet present in the limp penis. His body may be saying what his lips cannot. Such feelings are likely to be mixed with anxieties about his sexual powers.

Sexual difficulties following divorce are also quite common. Despite the release that divorce can bring there are always losses, some of which are recognized and acknowledged, while others are concerned with the loss of unconscious representations that the partner carried. For example, the search for a new partner can be fuelled by a hope of more rewarding sexual and emotional closeness, but the tendency to repeat relationship patterns that are unsatisfactory is strong. Sometimes a man who has chosen a more sexual woman this time round finds that his own interest wanes. It is as if the previous woman served a useful purpose by carrying his own projected lack of interest.

I want to pass on to the less obvious griefs that can affect sexual life, but first I must at least mention what is possibly the worst loss of all, the death of a child. It is hard for a parent to imagine how such a loss can be faced, and the pain can drive a wedge between the most loving of couples.

Luckily, the doctor is not alone in trying to provide comfort and support, and can call on the services of relatives, priests and communities. That is not to say that the doctor may not have specific tools that can be useful, particularly in helping people to talk about their bodies and sexual feelings at the same time that they are thinking of the lost child. Even as I write it feels in some way wrong, as if the juxtaposition of feelings of such profound loss with silly, sensual sexuality is shocking. Yet both spring from our deepest nature and cannot be separated.

Case Study 38

Mrs Hobbs was referred to a psychosexual doctor by the health visitor because she had not been able to make love for the last year, since her second baby was stillborn at 32 weeks. The lack of sexual life and the mutual loss for the couple was causing great strain in the relationship, and the first child was showing behaviour problems.

The patient was a very simple person and a Roman Catholic who believed that God lived in the sky. She began to tell the doctor about her love-making and said, 'You see doctor, when I begin to enjoy myself, I see the baby on the ceiling looking down and saying, "How can you enjoy yourself so soon after I am dead?"'

It has been said that one cannot work in a psychodynamic way with people who have a limited vocabulary. Such a view may be true for long-term, in-depth therapy, but the sort of body/mind work that I am describing here, which helps people to make connections within themselves, may well be possible. Indeed I learnt much from Mrs Hobbs, as she identified so clearly the exact moment, that is when she began to experience physical pleasure and arousal, that the block of grief and guilt turned her responses off.

The treatment was to liaise with the priest, who arranged a memorial service for the baby. There had been no ritual following the stillbirth, and Mrs Hobbs did not even know where the baby was buried. I must explain that my contact with this patient was many years ago and I am sure the loss would have been handled better now, but she has remained in my mind as a clear example of someone who, given an opportunity to talk, could link up her own emotions in a creative way. It had not been possible for her to explain to her husband why she was unable to make love, and he felt rejected and left to cope with his own grief unsupported.

Until it is possible to get in touch with one's own grief it cannot be shared or understood.

Case Study 39

Mrs James had been married for 2 years and had been unable to have an orgasm. She told the doctor that it was a happy marriage and that she loved her husband and wanted to be able to respond fully to him. She herself thought the problem was because she was very strictly brought up and her parents had been too shy to talk about sex. The doctor noticed that there was little emotion in the room and pointed out that the patient did not seem to have any strong feelings about the things she was mentioning. In response, and to her own and the doctor's surprise, she burst into tears and said, 'What I really care about is my first boyfriend who was killed in a car crash'. As soon as she had said it she wondered why, as she was sure she had put him behind her.

When she went home she was able to talk about the previous boyfriend with her husband, something she had never done before. He was sympathetic, did not appear to be jealous and comforted her in her renewed grief. This grief was fairly short-lived, as she truly did love her husband and was ready to put the past behind her. It seemed as though the fact of keeping the secret from her husband was at least in part the block to her arousal. She felt very close to him now she had shared such an important memory, and she was able to reach orgasm that night.

Two points need to be made about this case. The first is to warn against the danger of giving advice to patients about sharing secrets with their partner. Such openness may be helpful, as in this case, but the only person who is in a position to make that decision is the patient. In general terms frankness and discussion must be considered to be helpful in a relationship. In any particular instance many factors can limit the degree of openness possible. Advice along these lines may be slavishly followed, allowing a shift of blame onto the doctor when things go wrong. Alternatively, as with all advice given about the personal side of a patient's life, if the advice is ignored it may be difficult for the patient to come back and explain why. We forget the powerful position of the doctor in the imagination of patients at our peril and theirs.

Overly strict parents may help to create blocks in the sexual lives of their children, but they can also be used as scapegoats in the struggle to understand feelings that cannot be explained. Not everyone whose parents are strict gets into sexual difficulty, and it is more a question of the sort of relationship they have with that part of their parents that they have built into themselves that is relevant.

Many griefs related to fertility and childbearing can present as sexual problems. I have touched on the problem of separating sex from reproduction in Chapter 5 when discussing the Madonna/whore divide. For some women the ability to play with the idea of having a child is essential if they are going to be able to respond sexually. A most graphic example was a woman whose trigger for orgasm was to say to her husband, 'Give me a baby, give me a baby.' In reality she had four children and genuinely did not want any more, yet she needed to be able to use the phantasy. What a disaster it would have been had this woman been sterilized.

The sexual tensions produced by the strain of infertility, the investigations and the need to have intercourse at specific times have been well documented. Other losses are less easy to recognize.

Case Study 40

Mrs Knight, aged 39 years with one son of 8 years old, was taking the contraceptive pill and developed amenorrhoea. The doctor suggested that she should stop taking it and in due course did some hormonal tests. After two tests, she informed the patient that she was in the change. Mrs Knight sat silent and then left. Six months later she returned complaining that she was no longer able to enjoy sex. The doctor prescribed HRT, which made her feel better in herself but had no effect on her libido. When offered a longer appointment to talk more about it she began by discussing her next-door neighbour who had recently had a baby.

The doctor thought that they did not want any more children because she had used contraception for 8 years, but as the conversation continued it became clear that Mrs Knight had always planned to have another baby one day. When her first child was born they were in financial difficulty and had to accept that they could not afford another. Interestingly, the subject had not been discussed with her husband very much. She had always just assumed that they would have one when the time was right. The knowledge that she had reached the menopause at the comparatively early age of 39 years, with no warning signs, came as a bombshell to her.

At the time that this happened her sister's husband was diagnosed as having cancer, and it was difficult for Mrs Knight to accept that she had suffered any loss herself. It was as if, in the face of such grave news, there was no justification for her to grieve for herself, especially for what she felt to be an inadequate reason: 'After all, I have my son.' Yet she had lost what might have been several more years of fertile life, a time she had planned to put to good use. Several visits were needed before she could allow herself to feel the loss of the potential baby and mourn for it fully.

Other losses of part of the self include mutilating surgery such as mastectomy, hysterectomy or the making of a colostomy. Not only does the surgery affect the sense of body image and thus of self-esteem and attractiveness, but there is also the additional worry of how the partner now views the altered body. The loss of erotic response following his wife's mastectomy was a source of intense pain to one man, both for himself and for her, as he had loved her passionately.

It is often difficult for the couple to discuss the change in their physical life together, and both retreat into wordless solitude, which can be more painful than death itself. Main, in a discussion about the terminal care of a patient with cancer said, 'Cancer she could stand, but not this withdrawal of her husband'.[3] In relation to a woman complaining of loss of libido following the death of a baby, he pointed out that the death had happened several years previously and that it is often easier to talk about death than about sex. Cancer and death can be used as a defence against talking about sex. Buckman has some practical and sensible suggestions for patients and their carers about how to open up some discussion of the whole area.[4]

So far in this chapter I have written about the loss of loved ones, with examples of a father, grandmother, baby and former boyfriend. I have also mentioned the premature loss of fertility and the loss of physical health. Much is known about the mourning process,[5,6] and given a reasonably stable personality and the luck of supportive friends, relatives and professionals, there can be an expectation of recovery in due course.

When I think back over the patients that I and my colleagues have met, and when I reread the case vignettes in this book, I realize that it is often the more subtle losses that can act as a block to free sexual expression. I am reminded again of how false it is to try to separate emotions into finite categories as I have done here.

It is clear that for some of these patients the anxiety about their bodies represented a loss of some central sense of themselves as competent, whole people. For Miss Brooks (p. 12) the fear that the lump she had found in her vagina (her normal cervix) was a cancerous growth was so overwhelming that she suppressed it. Mrs Jones (p. 25) lost the sense of separate internal compartments following her uterovesicular fistula. I wonder what effect that had on her emotional representation of herself to herself. Did it create such a fear of fragility that a penetrating penis threatened total disintegration? Perhaps she was only able to keep a sense of wholeness by excluding any intrusion into her inner body or self. Certainly, after the initial 'moment of truth' when the body fantasy was revealed, she was unable to do any further work with the doctor. It was as though to allow the doctor to come closer to her feelings would be too much of a threat. At the time it had not occurred to the doctor to try to link the physical sensations to emotional ones. It may be that the sense of 'safe' compartments within, such as the womb, where things can be kept protected from dirty or destructive elements, needs to be explored further.

The loss may be of a fantasized perfect object or of some aspect of the future or the past. For Mr Daniels (p. 63), whose daughter was found to be taking drugs, it was not just the image of a happy, contented child with a bright future, but of himself as having been a satisfactory father. His fear that inadvertent physical contact had damaged her brought him face to face with his own fallibility and lack of perfection. For Mrs Rice (p. 64) the knowledge that her son was homosexual carried the sadness that he would not have a 'normal' family life. He would not be able to provide himself with children and herself and her husband with grandchildren. It was particularly difficult for her to accept and work through these losses because of her great love for her son and her abiding wish to accept him totally as he was.

For Mr Abbot, the first patient mentioned in this book (p. 6), the loss was of the precious sexual part of himself. It was difficult for doctors to sympathize with his feelings, for he projected the pain out of himself as impatience and fury with those who could not help him. For Mr King too (p. 26) his intense wish for a cure had provoked useless mechanical and surgical interventions. He dealt with the pain by dissociating his body from his mind in such a concrete way that the examining doctor could 'feel' a dividing line across the middle of him.

Finally, let me draw together three other stories from Chapter 8, in each of which there was a sense of vulnerability provoked by loss of control. Mr and Mrs Ball (p. 95) had embarked confidently on the experience of childbirth, but were suddenly threatened during the second stage of labour when things did not go entirely according to their plan. It was as if their ability to cope depended on a rigid exoskeleton that did not allow any bending or swaying in response to the winds of experience. Their uncertainties and fears could not be voiced and thus could not be worked through at the time in an appropriate emotional way. Instead they became fixed as a fantasized scar on her perineum.

For Mrs Z (p. 92) and Mr Edwards (p. 99) the need to be firmly in control of themselves and their outside worlds had arisen during childhood. Both had survived in the face of an unstable mother and absent father. Both had made a success of their professional life and married happily. However, for Mrs Z the earlier sense of vulnerability was reawakened when she was subjected to what felt like an attack from an older, uncaring, professional woman. The attack was felt within her physical body, the pain of the vaginal examination, but also on herself as a person by the comment that she had 'a low pain threshold'.

Mr Edwards had felt the reins of responsibility passed into his hands after his father died. (You may remember that at the age of 8 he was found planning to sell the house to secure the financial future for the family.) He had confidently handled those reins, with a lot of help from others, until he was suddenly faced by what seemed to be another life and death situation. He found himself alone in a room with his labouring wife, not understanding the process and convinced that she or the baby were going to die. He too was unable to talk about the feelings until he sought help for his impotence.

I am left with more questions than answers. What does it mean to the whole person to suffer such an overwhelming sense of loss of control? Perhaps for all of us there are experiences that arouse primitive fears of annihilation and death. For some these fears seem to be held at bay by particularly rigid control systems. If such a system is threatened, the hatches will be battened down as soon as possible and tighter than ever. Below decks the possibility of sexual arousal and release becomes locked away with the other feelings, and if there is no-one to help the individual find the courage to lift the lid, the sexual inhibition will remain, with all the secondary effects on the relationship and the family.

References

1   Murray Parkes C (1972) *Bereavement*. Tavistock, London.

2   Coombs J (1992) Loss of Libido. In *Psychosexual Medicine* (ed. R Lincoln), Chapman & Hall, London.

3   Main T (1987) In *Psychosexual Training and the Doctor/Patient Relationship* (ed. R Skrine), p 33. Chapman & Hall, London.

4   Buckman R (1988) *I Don't Know What to Say*. Macmillan, London.

5   Kubler-Ross E (1970) *On Death and Dying*. Tavistock, London.

6   Pincus L (1974) *Death and the Family: The importance of mourning*. Faber, London.

Part III
Making Connections

10

From the body to the mind

The title of the final section of this book came into my mind when a colleague asked, 'Which patients can you help? When does what you do work best?' I found myself answering, 'When I can help the patient make connections that he or she has not been able to make alone.' That is when, sometimes in a surprisingly short time, often during a consultation for some other problem, the doctor seems able to act as a catalyst that enables the patient to move forward. The connections made are most often between different parts of the individual: between the mind and the body, between some past memory and the present, between an emotion within and a sexual problem or physical symptom. Suddenly, more sense can be made of feelings and bodily pains.

Such revelatory moments are not very common, and much more of the work is concerned with muddling through with patients, tolerating not knowing what to do, offering a particular sort of doctoring for patients to use if they can. I have tried to demonstrate that sort of doctoring in the previous sections of the book. While writing, I have found myself wanting to read widely across different disciplines in order to try and make other connections, that is, to try to see where psychosexual medicine might lie in relation to other work. These two forms of connecting, that is, within the patient and between theoretical ideas and practical ways of doctoring, can be considered as two sides of the same coin. That coin has come into our possession as our cultural and professional inheritance and is imbued with the tradition of a body/mind divide.

The setting and the work

It has always seemed that the work described here crosses established borders between disciplines. Even in libraries and bookshops it is difficult to know in which section to put the books on the subject. Are they part of psychiatry? In terms of the number of psychiatrists who have become members of the Institute of Psychosexual Medicine, or have contributed to the literature,[1] one would not have thought so. Indeed the work described is not in the main with patients who would normally be part of a psychiatrist's workload. 'Apart from psychosexual difficulties our patients are managing their lives fairly well and can work at the doctor's pace'.[2]

Should it then be part of sexual therapy? That term has implications of behavioural or cognitive therapy. I suspect that ordinary doctors who have tried to develop these extra skills do allow some behavioural or cognitive responses to enter their work, perhaps to a greater degree than they realize and without always admitting it even to themselves. The underlying philosophy, however, is to try to think about the therapeutic relationship and to understand any lapses into advice-giving, reassurance or more directive teaching as an expression of the relationship at that moment. In addition to the different theoretical emphasis, many sexual therapists are not doctors, and the opportunity for the combined physical and mental approach is denied to those workers.

Because of the physical aspects of the work it does not sit comfortably with the psychotherapies, even though we may share some psychodynamic principles. We must recognize too that the training, based as it is on group work, with no insistence on personal therapy or personal supervision, provides a different level of interpersonal work. The responsibility of the body/ mind doctor to recognize those occasions when a more directive approach is necessary, indeed a central part of professional responsibility, as in the diagnosis and treatment of physical disease, means that the relationship with the patient, who is not a client, is bound to be very different from that of a psychotherapist. The length of treatment too, when offered in special consultations, is short, even when compared with so-called 'brief' psychotherapy, or episodic when a part of normal on-going medical care.

What then of other medical specialties? Many more gynaecologists and genitourinary specialists are recognizing that ailments are generated by the minds as well as the bodies of their patients and are seeking training to help them to consider the whole person in diagnosis and treatment.[3] Such an approach is particularly appropriate where patients have open access to the department, as in family planning and genitourinary medicine. Elsewhere, referral from a general practitioner often means that there is an obligation for the specialist to concentrate on physical illness and an assumption that the generalist doctor has made the decision that a physical opinion about a particular part of the body is required. That does not detract from the importance of a whole-person approach in hospital practice, but it does add complications for the doctor.

It seems that the logical place for psychosexual medicine is within general practice, where general practitioners have made important contributions to the work and form an appreciable percentage of the membership of the Institute. Yet it is still a small minority of such doctors who apply for and stick with even the basic 2 years of training. Despite this lack of interest in the training for themselves, a growing number value the availability of a specialist clinic where they can get help for their patients.

Such clinics have grown up in many areas as part of the family planning service, because that was where the work first originated, as was described at the beginning of this book. As community and hospital family planning is gradually becoming more integrated with gynaecology, the clinics are becoming more closely linked to those services. In many ways that seems appropriate, especially for our women patients. Some psychosexual doctors now work closely with urologists and andrologists, improving the service available for men. Yet neither of those settings is totally suitable. When running a psychosexual clinic in a gynaecology department I felt uncomfortable for my male patients who had to sit in the outpatients among the women, especially if they had come for personal help rather than as part of a couple. At that time the computer used in the department had no facility for recording them as male!

One further point about the provision of services should be made. In the past, when family planning was not considered respectable by the majority of the medical profession, the clinic was a rather private place, separate from general medical services, perhaps even rather hidden. Now the subject has become so respectable that it may be less easy for people to present what they feel are the less respectable parts of themselves. In Chapter 5 I discussed the feelings of shame and guilt that are so often a part of sexual feelings. It may be that more people now find the genitourinary clinic an easier place to which they can take the 'dirty' feelings they have about their sexuality. The tradition of particular confidentiality, enshrined in special legal provision, not only gives a sense of security, but also suggests a private atmosphere where the unspeakable can be spoken.

Another recent development within medicine and allied disciplines is the concept of sexual health. There are now sexual health clinics, where different aspects of sexual life can be considered as a whole. There must be many advantages to such a service, and I would not want to decry the thinking behind such a development. Yet there is something rather 'clean' about the idea of sexual health, and there are overtones of sex education and health advice. I do not for one moment argue with the idea that such education is necessary and important, but I am not sure how much it has to do with doctoring or understanding the real-life frailties of men and women. Education and the giving of information carry the implication that the educator knows best, that he has superior knowledge about what ails the patient and why. As

Bruno Bettelheim has said about his own introduction to psychoanalysis, 'We were equal in our efforts to learn significant things about me. This I found most reassuring, since it allayed my anxiety that things might be done to me without my knowing what they were ...'.[4]

I hope that doctors can leave much of the necessary education and information-giving to others, and create clinical situations in which they can interact with patients in an atmosphere of enquiry, and in which there can be a genuine search for a true understanding of the complicated bodily and emotional feelings that are present in the patient and in the consultation. Marinker has said that 'All the exciting things in the world happen on the boundaries',[5] and there is an exciting boundary to be explored between the body and the mind.

The need for theory – what theory?

Within the discipline of psychosexual medicine as it has developed in Britain since 1974, there has been an undercurrent of complaint that its practitioners should have more 'theory'. I want to pose the question of what theory, or theories, might be useful, and in what way they might affect the day-to-day practice of doctors and others.

My first concern is that the presence of theory in the mind of the practitioner will tend to fill up the 'space' between the two people. I have suggested that one or other of the participants to the consultation at times drops something into the space, perhaps a word such as 'hymen', perhaps a bodily reaction, that can then be processed and worked on by both people. Is it possible that the existence of theory in the mind would lead to an attempt to organize sensations and words too soon? Is it the lack of organization, the fact of not knowing, that allows a concentration on the here-and-now dynamics in the room? Perhaps the shared ignorance allows the making of connections that I believe are at the core of brief body/mind therapy. I am reminded of Peter Brook, writing about the production of plays, who says, 'In order for something of quality to take place an empty space has to be created ... If one doesn't search for security true creativity fills the space'.[6]

Let us think again about the way in which the work of the psychosexual doctor has developed. The seminar training system devised by Michael Balint and Tom Main was designed to increase the skills of doctors working in their normal settings, be that general practice, community clinics or hospitals. Because of the need for body/mind doctors and the perceived skills of some of these doctors, special psychosexual clinics were established.

All doctors running such clinics have a deep sense of inadequacy in the face of such far-reaching human distress. This feeling of not knowing is one of their strengths, for without theory to fall back on they have to try to stay with the ever-changing nature of the here-and-now relationship. However, we must recognize that some doctors have a greater talent for such work. For others, and I include myself among them, there is a constant pull to revert to easier ways of working. To reassure, to give advice, to cajole and to be satisfied with such behaviour without asking oneself, why?, why then?, what does my behaviour tell me about this person's problem?

In the face of such uncertainty there is a longing for theories that would provide reassurance. At the same time one must ask whether the absence of theory could be a rather self-satisfied belief that there is nothing useful to learn from others. Such is the view of some workers who have undertaken further training for themselves and found it useful.

If we believe that the sort of body/mind doctoring that I have been describing could be improved, how should we go about it? In a real world of finite time and energy we cannot expect every doctor to acquire and digest a knowledge of competing psychoanalytic theories in such a way as to be clinically useful. McDougall has said, in relation to psychoanalysis, 'Clinical elaboration involves a specific way of listening and trying to get into the patient's experience – a preoccupation with theory could only obscure what the analyst is trying to discern of the latest communication'.[7] Christopher, writing about her own experience of further training for psychosexual work says, 'All the trainings I have done are concerned to develop one's awareness and understanding of unconscious processes and communications and make them available to the patient'.[8]

Main has described two sorts of perceptiveness.[9] First is what he labels diacritic, 'concerning the capacity to perceive external events and to isolate, distinguish and intellectually manipulate ideas derived from external perception of the world around, treating facts and ideas as inanimate'. On the other side is what he calls co-anaesthetic or synaesthetic, which 'requires first, the operation of that part of the mind that is concerned not with logic or order but with the sense of oneself and others'. He considers that medical training is biased towards diacritic abilities, and one might see his work with the Institute of Psychosexual Medicine as an attempt to redress the balance. Yet he admits that each has its uses and its limitations.

Could we begin to think of our experience of body/mind doctoring in a diacritic light, that is, to organize and distinguish ideas, in such a way that we do not lose or interfere with the empathetic, feeling experiences of the clinical encounter? I believe that such theorizing might be possible, but it would have to grow out of the day-to-day work. Ideas from outside should not be imposed, but borrowed if and when, only when, they throw light on our work in our setting.

In a number of places in this book I have tried to do just that, as for example in my thoughts about the boundaries of the self and non-consummation (Chapter 6). This is a very tentative idea, and like any theory it is offered as a form of hypothesis to be tested against further experience.

In my search among other disciplines to try to find links that might stimulate the beginning of a theory of psychosexual medicine, I have been drawn to others who work with the body. Joan Chodorow, writing about dance therapy, says that it is based on the assumption that mind and body are in reciprocal interaction: 'In psychotherapy the two realms ... tend to split. By contrast a naturally felt emotion involves a dialectical relationship ... a union of body and psyche'.[10]

A dance therapist is, of course, working in a setting very different from that of a body/mind doctor, but the following passage produces echoes in my memory of times when patients have made sudden connections within themselves. 'When moving low close to the floor, an analysand suddenly remembered the full impact of what it was like when she fell and broke her leg at the age of six. In a seemingly random way, one of her legs had taken on a particular kind of twisted tension: the memory followed ... she remembered the painful, helpless, humiliating feeling when she tried to get up and could not. These were exactly the feelings that had brought her into analysis. She felt "unable to take a stand or stand on her own two feet".'

The author uses this as an example of an embodied link with the past. She says that in her psychotherapeutic practice she has 'felt it useful to keep feelers out for the fourfold crisis emotions: grief, fear, anger and contempt/ shame. More often than not the first three are named – the fourth is the missing one. Shame may be the hardest emotion of all to let ourselves feel.'

Can we find, in this description of her experience, a possible explanation for the potency of our work on some occasions, especially when related to the physical examination? Taking off one's clothes is such a revealing action, exposing those hidden areas of our bodies, laying ourselves open to the possibility of ridicule or disgust. Does the survival of such an experience give us the confidence to reveal other vulnerable feelings?

I am reminded of lecturing to continence advisers about sexual problems. From my own experience I emphasized the difficulty that most patients have in broaching the subject, the shyness and reticence, and the need for the professional to be sensitive. I was surprised when an experienced adviser said that patients often talked readily about sex, and as they explained it to me I suddenly felt a child in these matters: 'When a patient has had to discuss the intimate practical details, and has felt all the shame and horror of urinary and/ or faecal incontinence, sex is a comparatively easy and comfortable matter.' Now it occurs to me that the shame here may be dealt with by a collusive regression, which could make it hard for the patient to regain a more adult sexual privacy. I have certainly noticed a tendency to infantilize those who are incontinent, for example by delivering pads to the home when the patient was still mobile and could have collected them.

Returning to the question of theory in psychosexual medicine, Joyce McDougall says, 'Without the enrichment of self-knowledge theory is an impediment rather than an aid to what we hear'.[7] I have to wonder how much of the gain that is claimed by those who have had further training is as a result of theory and how much is from their own personal therapy? If our desire is to increase the interpersonal skills of the body/mind doctor, the personal experience of being listened to in a particular way might be more important than any theory. I know that my own ability to 'go in and feel, and pull out and think', that is, to develop an internal supervisor, has, almost without my realizing it, been enhanced by my personal psychoanalysis. The experience of having had internal, unknown anxieties recognized and voiced has made me more confident about voicing those which I feel in my patients. I do not claim that it has in any way trained me in psychotherapy, but it has helped me to be a more competent body/mind doctor.

Should we, therefore, in our search for theories about body/mind doctoring, look to those who can bring a greater understanding of themselves to the clinical encounter? It is my hope that more doctors who have had their own therapy will in the future remain working in this area of medicine, but there is a real difficulty. The fascination of the mind can be so great that doctors are tempted to move into psychotherapy or psychoanalysis, thus barring themselves from access to the body. Yet I believe that we are just at the beginning of an exploration of the everyday body/mind interactions that take place in all of us. If a group of doctors who continue to work in a body/mind way while having greater insight into themselves were to give their attention to matters of theory, we could perhaps begin to ask some pertinent questions.

At this point it may be useful to return to the idea of different structures of the personality, touched on earlier in the book. Samuels,[11] in discussing alternative imaginative structures, says, 'Does the psyche have to resemble a house, with foundations and upper stories?' Such an image carries inherent ideas of sequence, as though one stage followed another. He suggests that this view should be balanced by a concept of synchronicity, which sees the different aspects of the psyche as all being present simultaneously. He goes on to describe a numbering approach to states of mind, such as oneness, twoness and threeness. Main has said that the psychosexual doctor has to be able to work at a three-person genital level, with whole persons rather than part objects. This three-person relationship is seen in the ability to withdraw and observe the doctor and patient within the consultation, and also in the work with sexual problems, many of which are related to the three-person, Oedipal situation. Main continues, 'In distinction from psychoanalysis we can offer our patients little chance of developing and exploring infantile dependencies'.[2] While this is clearly so, because the limited time and training does not allow for the development of the necessary transference, I wonder whether longings and fears about separation and merging do not play a large part in sexual difficulties? Is there any way, in the setting in which we work, that such feelings are explored, at least to some degree? Perhaps our access to the body, the vulnerability of the physical examination, momentarily provides a sort of merging, with all that that implies of terror and satisfaction. Such an idea might explain those occasional moments of acute discomfort for the doctor when there is a sense that the patient's inner space has been invaded.[12]

We are left with the dilemma of what theory or theories to turn to in our search to understand what happens in these body/mind consultations. Although I do not find the counselling theories of Carl Rogers[13] very sympathetic or helpful to my work, he has interesting ideas about the place of theory. He says, 'There is no need for theory until or unless there are phenomena to explain ... there is no reason for a theory of therapy until there are observable changes which call for explanation ... the first requisite is a skill which produces an effective result.' Then, quoting Lawrence Henderson, he says, 'The physician must have first intimate, habitual intuitive familiarity with things; secondly, systematic knowledge of things; thirdly, an effective way of thinking about things.' I believe that we do now have some intimate familiarity with the work of body/mind doctoring, and that the time has come to try to find ways of thinking about what we do, but the problem of how to do so remains.

Bion has said that 'The trouble with theories is that they so soon make themselves out of date'.[14] We would not want to lift a half-digested theory from, say psychoanalysis, only to find that its practitioners have already moved on. Henrietta Moore, writing from a different discipline, suggests that anthropologists look for models to developmental theory, object relations theory, ego psychology and the work of Freud and Klein, but seldom to Lacanian or post-Lacanian theory, nor to any feminist theory.[15]

If, for example, we were to learn a Freudian view it would be challenged by feminists, who believe that patriarchal society creates women as feminine, showing the typical passive, masochistic and narcissistic characteristics.[16] Karen Horney is quoted as saying that women want to be men not because they are enamoured of the penis, but because men are in control of society.

I do not personally find the feminist psychoanalytic theory convincing, and what little I have tried to read about Lacan I find difficult to understand, but both views are part of the cultural and intellectual developments of our time and we cannot totally ignore them. However, I am not convinced that either view has specific relevance for psychosexual medicine. But neither can we hope to find a theory for our work by reaching back to an earlier system of thought and making it our own. What we find in practice is women who are in a great muddle about what it means for them to be women. I have met several people, both women and men, who have been bitterly disappointed when they have not been able to make their new ideologies work out in the practical setting of their relationships. Should we blame the fluid social and gender structure of the present day for their problems, or see such changes as a convenient receptacle for projected feelings from the person's internal world?

Recent work on the body/mind divide suggests that insights can be gained from systems theory. Human beings are conceived as being self-regulatory cybernetic systems, each comprising a hierarchy of subsystems that interface via the brain and with the larger social system.[17] Such a view suggests that 'the persistence of psychosomatic states and disorders in adults may be understood as remnants of arrests in affective development'.[18]

Another area of philosophical and linguistic research lays great emphasis on the notion of embodied experience. Mark Johnson, in his book '*The Body in the Mind*', describes 'the way in which our perceptual interactions and bodily movements within our environment generate schematic structures'.[19] He sees these image-schemata as extended in a metaphorical sense to reach beyond the physical to a non-physical, imaginative means of experiencing, understanding and reasoning about our world.

I find myself out of my depth in both systems theory and that of embodied experience, but I mention them to underline my concern that we do not try to find theories for our work by looking at those of any one discipline that is rooted in the past, without taking account of developing lines of thought elsewhere.

Where then can we start in our search for a theory to explain what goes on in psychosexual medicine and our efforts to conceptualize any ideas in a coherent fashion? Perhaps a possible place would be to go back to our patients and to the words they use when talking about their lives and pains.

References

1   *Bibliography*, Institute of Psychosexual Medicine, 11 Chandos Street, Cavendish Square, London, W1M 9DE.

2   Main T (1989) The Institute and Psychoanalysis: Debt, differentiation and development. In *The Ailment and Other Psychoanalytic Essays* (ed. J Johns), Free Association Books, London.

3   Editorial (1996) *Institute of Psychosexual Medicine Journal.* 12: 1.

4   Bettelheim B (1990) *Recollections and Reflections.* Thames and Hudson, London.

5   Marinker M (1986) Workshop in Research and Communication. *Institute of Psychosexual Medicine Newsletter.* 30: 7.

6   Brook P (1993) *There Are no Secrets.* Methuen, London.

7   McDougall J (1986) *Theatres of the Mind.* Free Association Books, London.

8   Christopher E (1996) Letter. *Institute of Psychosexual Medicine Journal.* 12: 2.

9   Main T (1989) Training for the Acquisition of Knowledge or the Development of Skills? In *The Ailment and Other Psychoanalytic Essays* (ed. J Johns), Free Association Books, London.

10 Chodorow J (1991) *Dance Therapy and Depth Psychology: The moving imagination.* Routledge, London.

11 Samuels A (1989) *The Plural Psyche.* Routledge, London.

12 Crowley T (1995) Seminar Training and the Development of Boundaries. *Institute of Psychosexual Medicine Journal.* 9: 6.

13 Rogers C (1951) *Client-centred Therapy.* Constable, London.

14 Bion W R (1990) *The Brazilian Lectures.* Karnac, London.

15 Moore H (1994) *A Passion for Difference.* Polity Press, Cambridge.

16 Tong R (1989) *Feminist Thought: A comprehensive introduction.* Unwin Hyman, London.

17 Taylor G J (1994) The Psychotherapeutic Application of a Dysregulation Model of Illness. In *The Imaginative Body* (eds A Erskine and D Judd), Whurr, London.

18 Stolorow R D and Atwood G (1991) The Mind and the Body. *Psychoanalytic Dialogues*. 1(2): 181–95.

19 Johnson M (1987) *The Body in the Mind: The bodily basis of meaning, imagination and reason*. University of Chicago Press, Chicago.

11

From the mind to the body

In the previous chapter I considered the setting in which the work of psychosexual medicine takes place and some possible theories that might be used to try to understand what goes on. None of the ideas seemed to be able to provide a totally appropriate basis within which to create a system of knowledge or an effective way of thinking about the work.

The use of language

One way of grounding our ideas in our day-to-day work is to study the language we use. In Chapter 3 I discussed the use of professional terms, some of which coincide with those of psychoanalysis, such as interpretation and projection, and others that we have specifically used in contradistinction, such as doctor–patient relationship rather than transference/countertransference. Another way to focus our work is to take notice of the words our patients use. Some words recur again and again, and seem to carry a particular emotional force. With experience the doctor can often produce a sense of empathy in the patient by the use of such a word at an appropriate time. I am thinking not just of what Chodorow calls the crisis emotions – grief, fear, anger and contempt/shame – but of words such as vulnerability and control, silliness, disgust and excitement, and of those which resonate within the body and mind, such as block, moistness, space and emptiness. Is it possible that such words might define the boundaries of a focused, brief therapy? I am not suggesting just a 'matching' of language, as is suggested by neurolinguistic programming, useful though that has been found to be.[1] My idea is rather that if we follow the words they may lead us into the specific areas of importance, and that from there we might reach out to make contact with other disciplines.

I believe it is important for us to develop a language in which the emotions that relate to the sexual body can be discussed both between doctor and patient and among doctors. The use of language borrowed from other disciplines is likely to alienate not only our patients, but our colleagues as well. If one reads Jungian psychology, terms such as 'puer', those characteristics associated with youth and creativity, and 'senex', those of the old man aspects of a person, can take on a useful meaning. For an outsider they leave one feeling excluded and lacking in understanding. The Freudian language of super-ego, ego and id formed a basis from which the working of the human psyche began to be studied, but ideas and languages have developed and diversified. Object relations theory, which underlies much psychotherapeutic understanding, is not easy for the newcomer to digest.

Post-modern philosophy suggests that we are formed by the language we use, and the Descartian view 'I think therefore I am' has given way to the Lacanian 'I think where I am not: therefore I am where I do not think.' Can we, within the language we find ourselves using with our patients and which they use with us, find some basis for a way to begin to systematize our knowledge and a more effective way of thinking about the experiences we have with them? Lane and Schwartz suggest that 'language is a means not only for representing experience (and implicitly its structure) but also for transforming experience'.[2] By grounding our thought within the clinical situation, while remaining open to what others have to offer, there may be ways of moving our understanding forward.

The concept of interpretation

As an extension or an example of these thoughts about language I find myself returning to the word 'interpretation' that was discussed briefly in Chapter 3. Psychosexual medicine shares this word with many of the psychotherapies, where it seems to be used with a variety of meanings. Different views are explored in a book edited by Hammer called *Use of Interpretation in Treatment: Technique and art*, published in 1968.[3] It has a slightly dated feel to it, but is nevertheless an interesting collection of very different views.

Garfield (Chapter 9) sees traditional interpretation as 'making conscious what was unconscious', and he suggests that this is different from focusing on the here-and-now behaving and experiencing. The word is used variously to describe the 'clarification of feeling' and 'the offering of an alternative view' (Chapter 1). Perhaps most importantly, a difference is made between the manner or style in which the comment is made and the content of the remark. It is suggested that the style is best if it is 'tender', although the content must be 'astringent'.

The 'depth' of the content is also discussed, and there is some agreement that it is the thoughts and wishes that are almost ready to emerge that need to be voiced by the therapist, and that the resistance to the material needs first to be recognized and interpreted. If not, the patient will not only deny the truth but feel attacked. Indeed, this fear that interpretations are threatening seems to lie behind the whole development of the Rogerian counselling school. Rogers is quoted as saying, 'Interpretations are usually threatening and tend to slow the speed and process of therapy' (Hammer, Chapter 1).

How do these various ideas relate to the work of psychosexual medicine? The central fact is that psychosexual work is of a particularly focused nature, concentrating on a small, although crucially important, area of the personality. It is concerned specifically with the feelings people have towards their bodies and towards the physical and emotional feelings of sexual arousal. Such feelings will, of course, reverberate at many different levels and in many different areas. In the brief therapy described in this book those reverberations are not explored explicitly by the doctor, although the opportunity to feel those echoes may allow the patient to make surprising connections. As has been stated, contact with the patient is brief or episodic, and the development of transference is not encouraged. In Chapter 9 of Hammer's book, Freud is quoted as saying that 'some degree of transference has to exist before interpretations could be offered effectively by the therapist'. We must therefore accept that the use of interpretation in brief body/mind work is different from that in long-term therapy.

In Chapter 21 of Hammer the function of therapeutic dialogue is said to be 'To raise the level of psychic organisation by naming the previously unnamed with words ... directing the patient's attention so that it will throw light upon a hitherto dark or hazy mental territory'. Such a description seems to me to apply particularly when we are trying to help a patient to find words for his or her ideas about the body. Those women who cannot allow anything into their vagina appear unable to conceptualize that area of their body in any way. Until they have the help of a doctor whom they feel knows about bodies, that part of themselves remains dark, unknown and unthinkable.

One of the points made by Hammer (in Chapter 22 of his book) is that visual imagery is a powerful tool to connect with feelings, and I am reminded of those patients who do not have the words with which to confront their fantasy with fact. Gradually, gropingly, they find some images, as has been demonstrated here. Ideas of 'a gate, curtains, a passage, a space, a void' rise into their consciousness. Such words must come from them, but the birth can be helped by the doctor who listens and does not impose his or her own image. The temptation to guess at the image by reference to those of other patients has to be resisted, so that something real for this patient can emerge in the space between them.

If such a space is created, the interaction between the doctor and patient is freed in ways that are not always easy to explain. Perhaps the concept of projective identification could be used to throw some light on what is going on, although the idea is a complicated one that has prompted much discussion.[4] It is based on an understanding and acceptance of the reality of unconscious phantasy and unconscious interaction. Ogden[5] explains that there are three stages to projective identification, which are taking place at the same time. First, the projector forces a part of himself into the other and uses it there to control him from within. Ogden makes the distinction between projection, in which the projector feels estranged from the other person, and projective identification, in which he feels at one with the person into whom he has projected part of himself. In the second stage the projector exerts pressure on the recipient to feel and act in a way congruent to the phantasy. An important point is that the projector is not trying to get rid of part of himself, but rather to keep it safe and live with it in another way. The third stage is the processing of the feelings by the recipient so that they can be taken back in a different and more manageable form.

I do not pretend to understand the ramifications of projective identification, and I am not sure how useful the concept may be to the body/mind doctor, who has often had no personal therapy and is not trained to use the less conscious part of himself. However, I feel in my gut that such unconscious transactions are of crucial importance to all human relationships. I suspect that it is often in action at those brief moments, particularly during the physical examination, when tensions and emotions are heightened and the consultation teeters on the brink of revelation or collapse.

Something about surviving the vulnerability of examination seems to allow a type of 'free association' within the patient. This phrase describes the classical psychoanalytic technique of asking the patient to say whatever comes into his mind. In practice such an activity is extremely difficult, because the habit of modifying and commenting on the thought almost simultaneously with its birth is present from the moment we acquire language and use it internally to talk to ourselves. To catch a thought on the wing takes much practice, and any attempt to suggest that someone should allow their mind to roam at the time of a physical examination would be unproductive, indeed unbearably threatening. All the doctor can do is to allow space and silence and remain absorbed in listening. Then connections may be made that surprise not just the doctor but the patient as well. Alternatively, of equal importance, there may be a total absence of any connection, as with Mr King

(p. 26), who seemed to have an almost physical line dividing his head from his genitals.

So far my remarks about psychosexual interpretation have been concerned with the physical examination of and ideas about the body. The other arm of the doctor's skill is the study of the changing relationship between the two people in the room. Despite all the limitations of a brief encounter, and of doctors who have only a limited understanding of their own internal worlds, it has been found to be possible to use an understanding of the relationship in such a way as to throw light on some aspects of the problems that patients bring to us. Again it may be the limited focus of the work, or the comparative stability of the patients treated in this way, that makes such interpretation possible.

We must not underestimate the power of the training method in sensitizing the doctor to the minute-by-minute changes during the consultation. Sometimes it is possible to discuss the defensive behaviour of the doctor who runs away into teaching, reassuring, prescribing or even sending for the partner. If the exact moment can be identified, it may illuminate the particular feeling within the patient and make it easier for the doctor to stay with and interpret the pain, anger or whatever when it surfaces on a future occasion. Sometimes it is even possible to interpret the evasive action. However, Samuels has said that he is not in favour of the 'that makes me feel' type of interpretation,[6] and we would hope that observations about the relationship would be used in a more indirect way. For example, the control that Mrs Carr (p. 33) exerted on the doctor was interpreted as her fear of loss of control, rather than as her ability to influence the doctor's actions.

It may be that the limited focus of the work in some way allows the doctor to become familiar with particularly potent interactions. Recurrent themes include that of the teacher–pupil relationship, where the patient's need to deny knowledge of sexual matters inveigles the doctor into supplying information or even drawing diagrams. In particular, those interactions based on the reality of the sex of the doctor can be a potent source of information on the feelings of the patient about his or her own sexuality.

Doctors are expensive people and they have to learn to use their time in an appropriate way. Many of us have come into the profession because of our own internal needs to feel liked and needed, and the temptation to just listen to a patient's story with sympathy must be resisted. Such a service can be offered by less expensive workers, and if we are to be worthy of our hire we must learn further skills, which I believe include the ability to listen, feel, think *and interpret* within the limits of our own work setting.

Malan describes the traditional areas of interpretation with the initials 'TOP', standing for transference, out there experiences in the patient's present life, and his past experiences. He also sees these aspects as a 'triangle of person', the present therapist, others in the present or recent past and parent.[7] A parallel 'triangle of conflict' has defence, anxiety and hidden feelings at its corners. The psychosexual doctor must, in my view, be aware of these areas of connection that the patient may make in order to be able to follow with empathy, and possibly facilitate the connection, but would not attempt to initiate such connections or claim any particular expertise in their interpretation.

The experience of body/mind doctoring suggests that there are specific ways in which some of the deeper areas of the psyche are reached, usually without the conscious design of the doctor. These areas are those in which the use of particular words, such as those suggested above, provide reverberations within the whole person. Although the doctor does not chase after any specific blocks based on preconceived ideas about the structure of the personality, patients often seem enabled to make their own connections. When they do they may be able to move on in their lives without further help, or they may decide to seek further psychotherapeutic help. At least the doctor then has the possibility of sharing in and offering comfort to a deeper pain.

I cannot leave this short foray into ideas about interpretation without quoting Christopher Bollas, who writes with such eloquence about his own experience of being an analyst.[8] He asks, 'What are the origins of an interpretation?' and suggests that 'The analytic space is somewhere between physical and psychic reality.' Later, 'Both patient and analyst ... rid themselves of such organisation of the unconscious in order to receive new unconscious communications, made possible through unknowing ... [this] establishes something of an essential dialectic, one that I think is at the heart of creativity in living, a dialectic between knowing (organising, seeing, cohering) and unknowing (loosening, no perceiving).' Do we, in our ordinary day-to-day doctoring, when we try to see the person as a whole, get a glimpse of this space between the psychic and physical reality?

Other brief therapies

I suspect that there is a lot that psychosexual doctors can learn from the experiences of those working in the brief psychotherapies. Alex Coren, working in a student counselling service, has much of interest to say about brief psychodynamic psychotherapy.[9] He points out that such an approach is often regarded as 'somehow an inferior and diluted version of the real thing ... much of the literature ... still appears to believe that the aim and purpose of short-term work is to convince the patient of the necessity for longer-term therapy'. His average number of sessions of around four is much closer to that of psychosexual medicine than it is to even brief focal psychotherapy, in which the usual number is quoted as anything from 15 to 30. He summarizes the sort of person who can be helped in brief therapy: 'a patient who is relatively healthy, well-functioning, with a well-defined area of difficulty'. Such a description corresponds in almost every detail to that of the patient suitable for brief psychosexual work.

However, we must recognize some of the many differences, not least the theoretical models that underlie the thinking of different workers. The psychosexual doctor already has a focus of work, that of the sexual or genital difficulty or pain. He has not been trained in longer-term therapy and does not therefore have to 'jettison all material not directly associated with the focus'. Because of the relative paucity of theoretical concepts and training he has, of necessity, to be guided by the patient and by the connections that he or she makes.

Coren's comments about not encouraging transference and the necessity for any working through to be done after therapy is finished are particularly apt for our work. Interestingly, he quotes Malan as saying that pre-Oedipal problems may be as amenable to short-term therapy as Oedipal ones.[10] I find that encouraging in view of my hypothesis that separation and dependence are often a factor in sexual difficulties. However, we may need to tread warily in that area if acute feelings of invasion and terror are to be avoided.

The advice that the question of ending should be around from the beginning is useful when a series of special meetings is offered by the doctor; in other words some sort of contract needs to be made. I believe that this is particularly important if the patient is trying to come to terms with loss of one sort or another, otherwise the unexpected ending may just reawaken old feelings of desertion without providing an opportunity for them to be worked through.

Other practical suggestions to therapists trained in long-term work may be less useful to traditional doctors. Such advice includes adopting a more questioning and confrontational style,[11] something that doctors have difficulty relinquishing in the first place!

Psychosomatic and psychosexual medicine

Much writing about psychosomatic medicine deals with those illnesses in which the psychological aetiology lies deeply within the personality, and where the origins can be traced back to the earliest times in the life of the individual. Any attempt at psychological treatment is assumed to be, of necessity, very long term. Yet McDougall, an analyst with great experience, particularly in relation to such deep-seated troubles as the sexual perversions,[12] says that 'We all tend to somatize at those moments when inner or outer circumstances overwhelm our habitual psychological ways of coping'.[13]

The patients whose clinical encounters are described in this book would not in the main be considered as suffering from psychosomatic afflictions of a profound type. Nevertheless, they are feeling their pains in an inappropriate part of themselves. In contrast to those people who seek help from a counsellor or psychotherapist, the patient who goes to a doctor with a sexual or physical symptom may not have considered the possibility of emotional help. Indeed, in many instances he would reject such help were it offered. The opportunity to make some connections within himself may be enough for him to move forward, or occasionally the experience of having been listened to and felt understood may give him enough confidence to seek further psychotherapeutic help.

Doctors and others are working to try to understand the interaction of body and mind at all sorts of different levels. '*The Imaginative Body*' is a collection of papers on the subject, and I was particularly interested in the chapter written by Dr Zalidis on the value of emotional awareness in general practice.[14] Yet he takes the decision to apply a psychotherapeutic approach in a very selective way, starting with an exhaustive history of the physical complaint. Here, I believe, he is trying to reach those deeper levels of psychosomatic dysfunction mentioned above. He seems to use either a physical or an emotional way of working. For the patients he is trying to help that may be necessary, although it implies a continuation of the body/mind divide.

The psychosexual doctor works differently, probably with a different group of patients. He works with what the patient brings and with what is happening at that moment in the room during discussion and during examination. He avoids history-taking as much as possible, although he also pays tribute to physical symptoms and does not deny their reality, even if no physical cause can be found.

This book has been written towards the end of the twentieth century by a doctor working in a Western democracy. Such temporal and social factors have to be taken into consideration when considering sexual matters and the attempts of all those who try to help people with sexual difficulties. The particular society in which men and women live exerts pressures on them in a number of obvious and less obvious ways. On behalf of my male patients, I cannot help feeling a twinge of envy for the ageing man in the fourth century BC who was not expected to perform sexually to any great extent.[15] The older man today is bombarded with articles and radio programmes dedicated to the idea that he can be helped to maintain his libido unchanged into his eighties. The message is not only that he can be helped to do so, with vacuum pumps and injections if necessary, but that somehow he *should* do so and that he is failing if he does not.

Let me end as I began, with an acknowledgment that sex is about minds and bodies. Older people are subject to all the emotional factors that have been discussed in this book, and many more besides, and an opportunity to discuss them may be welcome and helpful. At the same time one cannot deny that blood vessels and nerves may not be working quite as well as they were, and performance anxiety can be an additional complication. No-one wants to get old, or to lose such a precious and life-affirming activity, but this loss can be made worse if it is turned into a matter of personal failure. Secondary tensions between the couple can add to the misery, with the wife or partner feeling rejected, or that it is her fault that she is no longer attractive and desirable enough, or that she has become too powerful as their situations have changed.

The members of a partnership in which feelings have never been expressed easily, where perhaps the sexual act served as an important way of feeling close and understood, are particularly vulnerable to its breakdown. The fear of failure can make both people afraid of any cuddling or even affectionate touching, and they are left feeling isolated and desolate. If one partner is ill, the fear of causing damage may lead the other to withdraw sexually, without either of them realizing what the problem is or being able to talk about it. In our society, with its emphasis on youth, beauty and easy sex, the pain of ageing and loss of sexual prowess can be lonely and harsh.

It is the awareness of sexual unhappiness in the young and the old, and the effect that such distress can have on individuals and families, that has prompted doctors to search for better ways of helping. In this book I have tried to chart some of that search and to stimulate thought about how it might be continued. Helen Luke says 'As the great mystics have always known, we become what we look at, not that which we think about'.[16] How can we continue to look, both with our patients and at our work in general, yet not let ourselves get tied up by our thoughts? How can we avoid the thoughts about our practices, which I believe have some truly innovative aspects, from being turned into a hierarchy of ideas, yet encourage the development of a philosophy and theory of our subject?

To quote Samuels one last time, he cites Sullivan as saying, 'Inasmuch as you have problems to meet and solve, let me give you this pointer: Every problem contains and suggests its own solution'.[4]

If new work and new ideas are not to stagnate or regress, they must develop, and what I have been doing in the final section of this book is struggling to find a network, a web of ideas within which a theory of clinical work could evolve. To borrow a phrase from Adam Phillips,[17] I have been flirting with some possibilities. I have tried to suggest that there is a way forward that is neither a move further down the mainstream path of psychotherapy nor a regression into established physical doctoring roles of advice, reassurance or behavioural models of prescription. I now leave it for others interested in sexual problems to see whether they can find any strands in what I have written that they can pick up and unravel. I hope they can make their own connections so that we can further the understanding of human sexuality and the relationships between the body and the mind, and that in so doing doctors will continue to evolve skills to help those in trouble.

References

1   Clark A (1994) Neuro Linguistic Programming as an Aid in Psychosexual Counselling. *British Journal of Family Planning*. 20: 97–8.

2   Lane R D and Schwartz G E (1987) Levels of Emotional Awareness: A Cognitive–Developmental Theory and its Application to Psychotherapy. *American Journal of Psychiatry*. 144(2): 133–43.

3   Hammer E (ed.) (1968) *Use of Interpretation in Treatment: Technique and art*. Grune and Stratton, Sidcup.

4   Sandler J (ed.) (1988) *Projection, Identification, Projective Identification*. Karnac, London.

5   Ogden T (1979) On Projective Identification. *International Journal of Psycho-Analysis*. 60: 357.

6   Samuels A (1989) *The Plural Psyche*. Routledge, London.

7   Malan D (1979) *Individual Psychotherapy and the Science of Psychodynamics*. Butterworths, London.

8   Bollas C (1989) *The Forces of Destiny: Psychoanalysis and the human idiom*. Free Association Books, London.

9   Coren A (1996) Brief Therapy; Base Metal or Pure Gold? *Psychodynamic Counselling*. 2(1): 22–38.

10   Malan D (1992) *Psychodynamics, Teaching and Outcome in Brief Therapy*. Butterworth Heinemann, London.

11   Bauer G P and Kobos J C (1987) *Brief Therapy: Short term psychotherapeutic intervention*. Jason Aronson, London.

12   McDougall J (1995) *The Many Faces of Eros*. Free Association Books, London.

13   McDougall J (1989) *Theatres of the Body*. Free Association Books, London.

14   Zalidis S (1994) The Value of Emotional Awareness in General Practice. In *The Imaginative Body* (eds A Erskine and D Judd), Whurr, London.

15   Foucault M (1992) *The History of Sexuality*, Vol. 1. Penguin, London.

16   Luke H (1992) *Kaleidoscope*. Parabola Books, New York.

17   Phillips A (1994) *On Flirtation*. Faber and Faber, London.

Index